# Practical Guide for Pain Interventions: Head and Neck Sonoanatomy

Taylan Akkaya • Ayhan Cömert
Editors

# Practical Guide for Pain Interventions: Head and Neck Sonoanatomy

Springer

*Editors*
Taylan Akkaya
Etlik City Hospital, Department
of Anaesthesia and Pain Medicine
Ankara, Turkey

Ayhan Cömert
Ankara University School of Medicine,
Department of Anatomy
Ankara, Turkey

ISBN 978-3-031-88772-7 ISBN 978-3-031-88773-4 (eBook)
https://doi.org/10.1007/978-3-031-88773-4



This Springer imprint is published by the registered company Springer Nature Switzerland AG
The registered company address is: Gewerbestrasse 11, 6330 Cham, Switzerland

# Contents

# Sonoanatomy in Pain Practice

Cüneyt Yücesoy, Z. Banu Aydın, Taylan Akkaya, and Ayhan Cömert

## Introduction

Ultrasound (US)-guided nerve blocks are useful techniques in pain management for physicians to learn. In previous years, traditional procedures in pain medicine were performed using anatomic landmarks, fluoroscopy, or computed tomography (CT) [1]. The procedures in pain medicine practice necessitate image guidance for accurate, safe, and diagnostic interventions.

Fluoroscopy relies on the bony landmarks without visualization of the soft tissues, such as the spinal cord, nerves, vessels, ligaments, tendons, and muscles in the region of interest. The US is free of radiation risk against CT and fluoroscopy. It is portable, cost-effective, and allows direct real-time visualization of soft-tissue structures. It has become a common practice to use US guidance in chronic pain management procedures in musculoskeletal systems, peripheral, and neuraxial pathologies [1, 2]. However, it is operator-dependent and requires training and practice to gain expertise about all available transducers, technologies, and possible frequencies for the proper imaging. Today, US-guided nerve blocks are routinely used in regional anesthesia practice in many centers around the world [3, 4].

Real-time US images are integrated images that result from reflection from organ surfaces and scattering into heterogeneous tissues. The most important step for success in US-guided nerve blocks is the optimization of the US image. The US allows real-time visualization of various tissue structures, including muscles, tendons, ligaments, nerves, vessels, and bone surfaces, and additionally visualization of needle advancement and the spread of the injected material [5]. US-guided needle insertion and drug administration provide an advantage in ensuring accuracy and avoiding complications such as injury to the nerve and vascular structures [6]. Also, the US provides good visualization of bony surfaces. With the advances in US technology the view of small peripheral nerves and their associated branches is possible [7]. Superficial spine interventions such as medial branch block, facet intra-articular injections, and nerve root blocks can be visualized with US [3]. However, structures hidden by bone cannot be visualized well, because

C. Yücesoy
Duzen Laboratories Group, Radiology Department, Ankara, Turkey

Z. B. Aydın (✉)
Hitit University Faculty of Medicine, Department of Radiology, Çorum, Turkey

T. Akkaya
Etlik City Hospital, Department of Anaesthesia and Pain Medicine, Ankara, Turkey

A. Cömert
Ankara University School of Medicine, Department of Anatomy, Ankara, Turkey



T. Akkaya, A. Cömert (eds.), *Practical Guide for Pain Interventions: Head and Neck Sonoanatomy*,
https://doi.org/10.1007/978-3-031-88773-4_1

bone has a high attenuation coefficient and creates an acoustic shadow. The other limitations of US usage are obesity and deeply situated structures. Visualization of deeper structures requires the use of a low-frequency curvilinear probe. While this allows viewing of deeper structures, it distorts the resolution.

Various types of US-guided interventional pain procedures include neuraxial (facet joint blocks, medial branch nerve blocks, epidural injections, etc.), intraarticular (knee, wrist, elbow, shoulder, etc.), peripheral neural (stellate ganglion, greater occipital nerve, branches of brachial plexus, etc.) injections, and myofascial trigger points injections [8]. Additionally, radiofrequency treatments, providing longer-lasting effects, can be performed successfully using the US. In the head and neck, the US has an expanded role in guidance of the neural interventional procedures, and main US-guided pain interventions such as trigeminal and occipital nerve blocks, selective cervical root blocks, cervical facet and medial branch blocks, cervical sympathetic blocks, sphenopalatine and glossopharyngeal nerve blocks, and myofascial trigger point injections can be applied successfully by experienced physicians. In patients suffering from neck pain, the sonographic visibility of the cervical medial branches is important to identify the responsible joint and for the diagnostic blocks of the cervical medial branches. Eichenberger et al. reported the visualization of the third occipital nerve using the US and accurate blockage with local anesthetic under US imaging [9]. In occipital neuralgia, US guidance allows precise occipital nerve blocks and interventions at the level of the specific location [10]. Great occipital nerve blocks with local anesthesia can aid in the diagnosis and treatment of occipital neuralgia and have shown efficacy in the diagnosis and treatment of cervicogenic headaches [11]. Galiano et al. studied the feasibility of the US as a guiding tool for simulated cervical facet joint intra-articular injections in cadavers [12]. Also, using US imaging is applicable to guide the selective cervical nerve root blocks [13, 14]. Narouze et al. performed cervical nerve root block under US imaging as the primary imaging tool, and with fluoroscopy as the control, in their study of ten patients [14]. The US allows the real-time visualization of the spinal nerves and vessels and improves the safety of the technique [14]. Blockage of the branches of the trigeminal nerve in the pterygopalatine or infratemporal fossa is traditionally performed using an image-guidance approach of either fluoroscopy or CT [15]. In addition, US guidance allows the visualization of the vessels, such as the maxillary artery, and is also successful in trigeminal nerve blockage [15]. Local anesthetics injected into the pterygopalatine fossa are expected to anesthetize the trigeminal ganglion, pterygopalatine ganglion, maxillary nerve, and mandibular nerve by the spread of the injectate to the infratemporal fossa and the Meckel's cave [16]. Cervical plexus blocks can be performed more safely and accurately under US guidance, facilitating the identification of various landmarks including muscles, cervical vertebrae, large vessels, nerves, and the cervical fascia [17]. Additionally, cervical sympathetic and stellate ganglion blocks can be applied under a US-guided approach and provide a valuable diagnostic and therapeutic benefit to sympathetically maintained pain syndromes in the head, neck, and upper extremities [18].

## Conclusion

US utilization for pain interventions increases in practice due to its real-time identification of target structures, needle placement, and visualization of therapeutic medication. Furthermore, it provides radiation-free experiments both for the physician and the patient. Ultrasonographic visualization of nerves requires excellent anatomical knowledge and experience. The major limitations of the US include artifacts caused by bone structures and decreased resolution in deep structures and obese patients, leading to challenges in nerve identification. Adequate training is mandatory before the US is used for pain intervention, especially pain medicine in the head and neck, where the neural and vital soft tissue structures and vessels are compacted in a limited area. The field of pain medicine continues to evolve through new literature, advanced sonoanatomy information, and sharing of experiences.

## References


1. Li J, Szabova A. Ultrasound-guided nerve blocks in the head and neck for chronic pain management: the anatomy, sonoanatomy, and procedure. Pain Physician. 2021;24(8):533–48.
2. Akkaya T, Alptekin A, Özkan D. Ultrasound-guided chronic pain interventions (part II). Agri. 2016;28(2):59–66.
3. Narouze SN. Ultrasound-guided interventional procedures in pain management. Reg Anesth Pain Med. 2010;35(2):55–8.
4. Narouze SN, Provenzano DA. Sonographically-guided cervical facet nerve and joint injections: why sonography? J Ultrasound Med. 2013;32(11):1885–96.
5. Bhatia A, Brull R. Is ultrasound guidance advantageous for interventional pain management? A systematic review of chronic pain outcomes. Anesth Analg. 2013;117(1):236–51.
6. Soneji N, Peng PWH. Ultrasound-guided pain interventions – a review of techniques for peripheral nerves. Korean J Pain. 2013;26(2):111–24.
7. Suk JI, Walker FO, Cartwright MS. Ultrasonography of peripheral nerves. Curr Neurol Neurosci Rep. 2013;13(2):328.
8. Korbe S, Udoji EN, Ness TJ, Udoji MA. Ultrasound-guided interventional procedures for chronic pain management. Pain Manag. 2015;5(6):465–82.
9. Eichenberger U, Greher M, Kapral S, Marhofer P, Wiest R, Remonda L, et al. Sonographic visualization and ultrasound-guided block of the third occipital nerve: prospective for a new method to diagnose C2-C3 zygapophysial joint pain. Anesthesiology. 2006;104(2):303–8.
10. Narouze S. Occipital neuralgia diagnosis and treatment: the role of ultrasound. Headache. 2016;56(4):801–7.
11. Pingree MJ, Sole JS, O' Brien TG, Eldrige JS, Moeschler SM. Clinical efficacy of an ultrasound-guided greater occipital nerve block at the level of C2. Reg Anesth Pain Med. 2017;42(1):99–104.
12. Galiano K, Obwegeser AA, Bodner G, Freund MC, Gruber H, Maurer H, et al. Ultrasound-guided facet joint injections in the middle to lower cervical spine: a CT-controlled sonoanatomic study. Clin J Pain. 2006;22(6):538–43.
13. Galiano K, Obwegeser AA, Bodner G, Freund MC, Gruber H, Maurer H, et al. Ultrasound-guided periradicular injections in the middle to lower cervical spine: an imaging study of a new approach. Reg Anesth Pain Med. 2005;30(4):391–6.
14. Narouze SN, Vydyanathan A, Kapural L, Sessler DI, Mekhail N. Ultrasound-guided cervical selective nerve root block: a fluoroscopy-controlled feasibility study. Reg Anesth Pain Med. 2009;34(4):343–8.
15. Nader A, Kendall MC, Oliveria GS, Chen JQ, Vanderby B, Rosenow JM, et al. Ultrasound-guided trigeminal nerve block via the pterygopalatine fossa: an effective treatment for trigeminal neuralgia and atypical facial pain. Pain Physician. 2013;16(5):537–45.
16. Nader A, Schittek H, Kendall MC. Lateral pterygoid muscle and maxillary artery are key anatomical landmarks for ultrasound-guided trigeminal nerve block. Anesthesiology. 2013;118(4):957.
17. Saranteas T, Paraskeuopoulos T, Anagnostopoulou S, Kanellopoulos I, Mastoris M, Kostopanagiotouet G. Ultrasound anatomy of the cervical paravertebral space: a preliminary study. Surg Radiol Anat. 2010;32(6):617–22.
18. Narouze SN. Ultrasound-guided stellate ganglion block: safety and efficacy. Curr Pain Headache Rep. 2014,18(6).424.

# Ultrasound Imaging and Guidance: Gauging Musculoskeletal Interventions

Levent Özçakar, Vincenzo Ricci, and Murat Kara

According to the EURO-MUSCULUS/USPRM global report [1], ultrasonography is used much more commonly for diagnostic (than interventional) purposes. While this is at least true for academic production, the actual scenario in musculoskeletal (MSK) practice might significantly vary among centers—especially for those who (underestimate the diagnostic side of the story and) dive into interventional procedures with the support of ultrasound (US) guidance. Seemingly, such colleagues also consider the lengthy education of MSK US to be shorter/easier for the interventional side [2, 3]. Without extra discussion on these "vague" issues in this chapter, we wish to draw attention to the concomitance/balance of the two aforementioned concepts [4]. Accordingly, we will be homing in on philosophy as well.

Owing to its several advantages, MSK US is already accepted as more than an imaging tool—and rather as the continuation of physical examination in daily practice [5]. Moreover, for innumerous reasons [6, 7], it is also perceived as the "X factor" for MSK clinicians [8]. Herein, it would be noteworthy that the first rule/step in MSK US is "seeing is believing" [9]. The second/third rule(s) would be "if you can see it, you can describe/quantify it and you can have access to it" [4]. The latter serves as the main denominator of interventional US and also replies to the other/common question, i.e., "Which imaging tool should I use for guiding a particular procedure?". In other words, if the US can show a structure/pathology because of its high resolution, it is the imaging tool of choice for diagnostic and interventional purposes alike. On the contrary, again due to well-known reasons [10], if US cannot show a structure/pathology; it is—for sure—not "on the table" as an alternative.

To this end, also sufficing with the clarity on the role of US for interventional precision, we wish to further the discussion as regards clinical decision-making before the procedure. Regardless of the imaging tool used for the diagnosis or the physician who had initially established the diagnosis (usually the same person in the case of US-oriented MSK physicians), US significantly contributes to the decision-making process [11]. Likewise, we imply that the US "guides the whole procedure" rather than simply partaking in needle follow-up [12]. To be more specific, the US examination can (even) refrain from

L. Özçakar · M. Kara
Hacettepe University Medical School, Department of Physical and Rehabilitation Medicine, Ankara, Turkey

V. Ricci (✉)
Physical and Rehabilitation Medicine Unit, Luigi Sacco University Hospital, ASST Fatebenefratelli-Sacco, Milan, Italy



T. Akkaya, A. Cömert (eds.), *Practical Guide for Pain Interventions: Head and Neck Sonoanatomy*,
https://doi.org/10.1007/978-3-031-88773-4_2

an intervention and can help to ascertain the target or where/what/how to inject. Should the patient undergo surgery, it can also provide indirect navigation for the surgeon as well as direct guidance during minor surgeries [4]. Finally, close/optimal follow-up after the procedure(s) can indisputably be possible with the US. Herein, a side note would be the possible contribution of the US within the concept of "sono-feedback" [13]. We wish to remind that the use of US is patient- and physician-friendly. As such, by sharing the static/dynamic images on the screen with the patient, it is possible to naturally involve the patient in the examination/procedure. Indeed, the treatment outcome has been shown to positively change in such cases [13]. In the past, physiatrists were classifying the word US as (diagnostic) ultrasonography and (therapeutic) deep heating modality. However/ironically, in current practice, diagnostic US can also be considered "therapeutic" in the hands of expert physician sonographers.

At this point, it would perhaps be sound/necessary to say a few words on the interventional technique. Before, the majority of the procedures were being performed using anatomical/superficial landmarks, i.e., referred as "blind" techniques. In this sense, senior colleagues who have previously used such blind methods (but who also/later adopted US guidance) unintentionally develop "ambiguous" skills. Interestingly, they sometimes/still need to touch a bony target despite their target being a soft tissue nearby. Herein, junior colleagues who are "born and bred" with the US (imaging and guidance) therefore seem to be advantageous.

Last but not least, we wish to also/partially object to the discussion of whether US guidance improves the treatment outcome when compared with blind techniques. Yet, the pertinent literature comprises several articles in favor and against, whereby the comparison is usually done using either certain pain or functional assessments. Herewith, data concerning how many structures are being injured (or endangered) during the procedure are not/never compared, i.e., apples and oranges?

In closing, we imply that US imaging and guidance are equally contributory during the whole procedure in myriad interventions. Physicians must see in advance to bethink where/what/how to inject, and, depending on their expertise, they can freely choose the best approach to intervene (Fig. 1). Of note, the US is like glasses, and, within the dilemma of liberty versus threat [14], the person who uses them needs to decide whether/where to take them off.

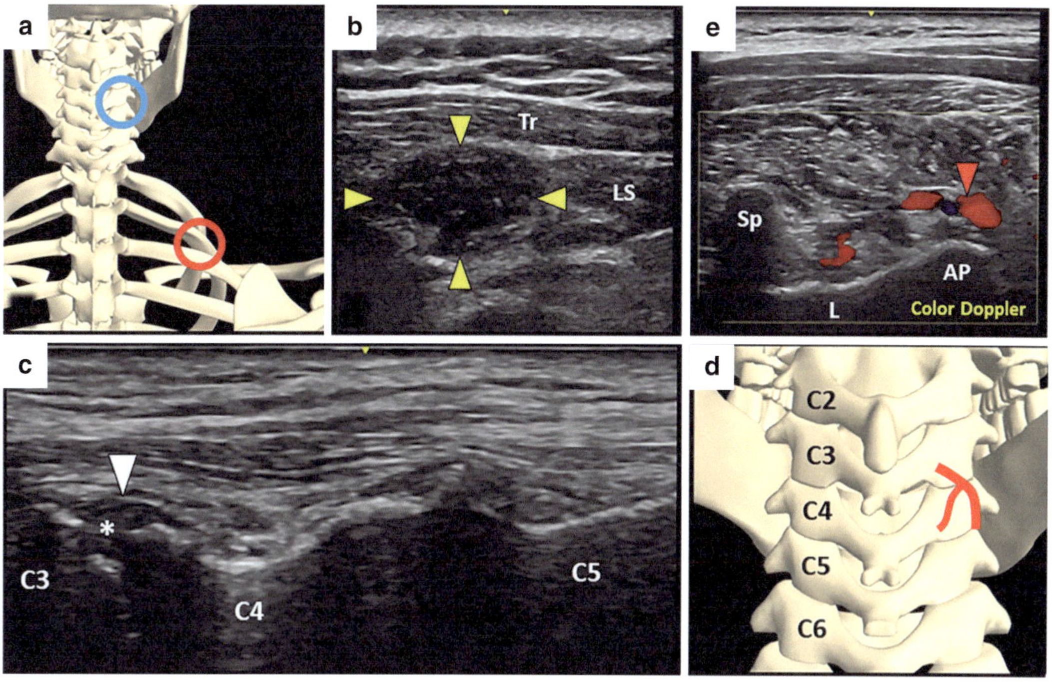


**Fig. 1** Navigating with Ultrasound Through the Complexity of Cervical Pain. Two different painful spots—along the cervical spine *(blue circle)* and proximal to the right scapula *(red circle)*—have been manually identified during the physical examination of a patient with cervical pain (**a**). Sonographic examination revealed a large myofascial trigger point *(yellow arrowheads)* in the levator scapulae muscle *(LS)* close to the edge of the right scapula (**b**) and osteoarthritis of the right C3–C4 facet joint *(white arrowhead)* with intra-articular effusion *(white asterisk)* (**c**). Rotating the probe at 90° to accurately plan for an US-guided procedure in the proximal cervical spine, vascular elements *(red arrowhead)* have been identified nearby the right C3–C4 facet joint, on the commonly used needle pathway to inject this joint (**d**, **e**). Note that the US promptly "guides" the physician for both identification of the pain generators and planning safe interventions. Tr trapezius muscle, red lines: vessels, Sp spinous process, L lamina, AP articular pillar

**Author Disclosures** Conflict of interest: None. No funding was received.

## References

1. Kara M, Gürçay E, Ekiz T, et al. EURO-MUSCULUS/USPRM global report on musculoskeletal ultrasound publications. Am J Phys Med Rehabil. 2020;99:847–52.
2. Wu WT, Chang KV, Han DS, et al. Musculoskeletal ultrasound workshops in postgraduate physician training: a pre- and post-workshop survey of 156 participants. BMC Med Educ. 2019;19:362.
3. Foti C, Ozçakar L, Kara M, et al. Changing the awareness of physiatrists on musculoskeletal ultrasound: Italy in EURO-MUSCULUS. Int J Rehabil Res. 2013;36:178–81.
4. Levent Ö, Franco F, Vincenzo R, Ke-vin C, Gürçay Eda PG, editors. Ultrasound imaging and guidance for musculoskeletal interventions in physical and rehabilitation medicine. 1st ed. Milan: Edi-ermes; 2020. p. 192–6.
5. Ricci V, Özçakar L. From "ultrasound imaging" to "ultrasound examination": a needful upgrade in musculoskeletal medicine. Pain Med. 2020;21:1304–6.
6. Özçakar L, Kara M, Chang KV, et al. Nineteen reasons why physiatrists should do musculoskeletal ultrasound: EURO-MUSCULUS/USPRM recommendations. Am J Phys Med Rehabil. 2015;94:e45–9.
7. Özçakar L, Ricci V, Chang KV, Mezian K, Kara M. Musculoskeletal ultrasonography: ninety-nine reasons for physiatrists. Med Ultrason. 2022;24:137–9.
8. Ricci V, Özçakar L. Ultrasonographic examination: the "x-factor" in physiatry. Am J Phys Med Rehabil. 2020;99:e131–2.
9. Cauvin ER. Musculoskeletal ultrasonography: seeing is believing. Vet J. 1999;158:4–5.
10. Özçakar L. Sonographic atlas for common musculoskeletal pathologies. Milan: Edi Ermes; 2017. ISBN: 9788870515763

11. Özçakar L, Onat ŞŞ, Gürçay E, et al. Are blind injections ethical or historical?: think twice with ultrasound. Am J Phys Med Rehabil. 2016;95:158–60.
12. Sekizkardeş M, Aydin G, Özçakar L. Ultrasound-guided shoulder injection or ultrasound guides the shoulder injection? Standard versus state-of-the-art. Am J Phys Med Rehabil. 2018;97:e46.
13. Çağlayan G, Özçakar L, Kaymak SU, et al. Effects of sono-feedback during aspiration of baker's cysts: a controlled clinical trial. J Rehabil Med. 2016;48:386–9.
14. Özçakar L, Ekiz T, Aydin G, et al. Musculoskeletal ultrasound "threatening"physical and rehabilitation medicine: a prime caution regarding foxes. Eur J Phys Rehabil Med. 2018;54:499–500.

# Basic Principles in US Imaging and Sectional Anatomy

Uğur Toprak and Ayhan Cömert

## Basic Principles and Physics of Ultrasound

Ultrasound is sound at a frequency (>20.000 Hz) higher than that of the range of human hearing (20–20.000 Hz). In diagnostic ultrasound, which is used for the evaluation of internal structures, sound waves pass through a transducer to the body, and the non-absorbable part of tissues is scattered or reflected. Echoes returning to the transducer are coded according to their frequencies, producing the image of these structures.

A sound wave is a mechanical energy that travels in a conductive medium, consisting of regions of high and low pressure, i.e., sound requires a material medium for propagation; it does not move through the vacuum. The properties of a sound wave are explained by the parameters of pressure, wavelength, frequency, period, and velocity (Fig. 1).

Wavelength ($\lambda$): The spatial period of the sound wave determined by measuring the distance between two successive points of the same phase. It is expressed in meters ($m$).

Amplitude ($A$): A measure of the wave height expressed in meters ($m$).

Period ($T$): The time it takes for one full wave cycle to occur, expressed in seconds.

Frequency ($f$): The number of cycles completed per second. Wavelength ($\lambda$) is inversely proportional to frequency ($f$). The unit of frequency is hertz (Hz).

Velocity: The speed of propagation of a sound wave in a medium (m/s). It is the product of frequency ($f$) and wavelength ($\lambda$).

Energy ($E$): The energy of the sound wave is proportional to the square of its amplitude ($A$); i.e., as the amplitude of the wave decreases (as it penetrates deeper), the energy carried by the wave decreases to a great extent.

Power ($P$): The energy ($E$) transmitted per unit time ($t$).

The speed of sound varies according to the environment. While it is 330, 1.430, and 5.000 m/s in air, pure water, and metal, respectively, it is 1.450, 1.550, 1.570, 1.585, and 4.080 m/s in fat, liver, blood, muscle, and bone, respectively. In soft tissues, this value is considered to be 1.540 m/s on average [1].

Today, transducers have artificial crystals, which use the piezoelectric principle to produce sound waves in ultrasound. Materials used in crystals produce voltage when deformed by the applied voltage or pressure, which is called piezoelectricity. Thus, electrical energy is con-

U. Toprak (✉)
Eskisehir Osmangazi University, School of Medicine, Department of Radiology, Eskisehir, Turkey

A. Cömert (✉)
Ankara University School of Medicine, Department of Anatomy, Ankara, Turkey


T. Akkaya, A. Cömert (eds.), *Practical Guide for Pain Interventions: Head and Neck Sonoanatomy*, https://doi.org/10.1007/978-3-031-88773-4_3

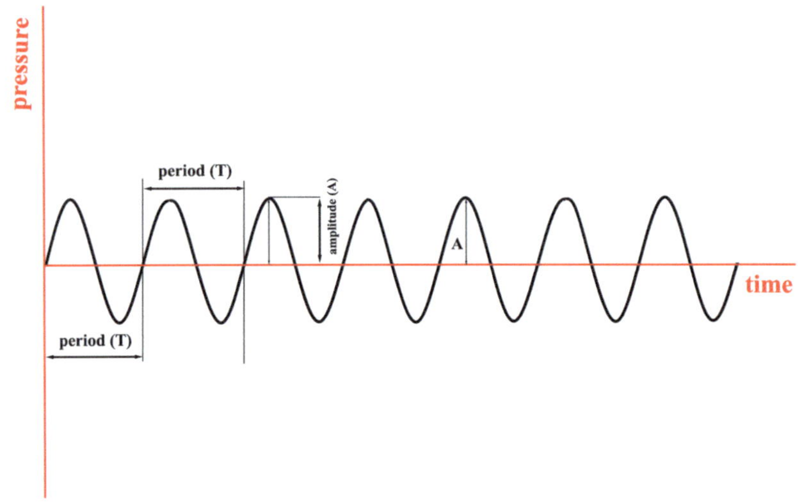


**Fig. 1** Presentation of ultrasound waveform

verted into sound waves (mechanical energy) and sent to the tissue, and sound waves returned by the tissue are converted back into voltage and analyzed by the system.

Very short pulses are required to produce diagnostic ultrasound images; therefore, the ringing of the crystal is soon stopped by damping material applied to absorb the vibrations. Thus, ultrasound waves are produced in pulses. Each pulse usually consists of two or three sound cycles of the same frequency. The pulse repetition frequency (PRF) is the number of pulses emitted by the transducer per unit time. Ultrasound pulses should be placed at sufficient time intervals to allow the sound to reach the target and return to the transducer before the next pulse is generated. For diagnostic imaging, PRF ranges from 1 to 10 kHz.

An ultrasound transducer has dual functions: the production of ultrasound waves and the reception of the waves reflected from the tissues after a certain period of time. This is known as pulse wave ultrasound. Simply, a basic transducer consists of three parts: (1). case, (2). crystal, and (3). damping material. The transducer is connected to the ultrasound system with an electrical cable. Most real-time transducers use many small crystal elements to generate each pulse.

The transducer to be selected changes depending on the depth of the structure desired to be visualized. If superficial tissues are to be examined, a high-frequency transducer with low penetration should be preferred, while a low-frequency transducer with high penetration is suitable for the examination of deep tissues. The higher the frequency, the higher the resolution. Linear transducers are utilized to evaluate superficial structures, such as the neck and thyroid. The frequencies of these transducers generally vary between 7 and 15 MHz, and their penetration is limited to 2–3 cm. Convex transducers are preferred to evaluate thicker, deeper tissues (such as the abdomen and pelvis). At a frequency ranging from 2 to 5 MHz, they achieve approximately 4–5 cm of penetration through the skin. Lastly, microconvex transducers are used in tissues where deep penetration is targeted through a small acoustic window, such as the heart.

## Basic Functional Features of the Ultrasound Device

In order to obtain an optimal ultrasound image, it is necessary to know the basic functions of the device.

### Gain

Echoes returning from tissues reach the crystals and produce an electric current, from which an image is obtained. Each bright pixel is then converted into an image, proportional to the energy of the returning wave. However, due to the very small amplitude of the returned echo signals, amplification is needed. The amplification of the signal can be adjusted using the "gain" control, but using this function contributes to the background noise. Excessive increase in gain may hide minor changes in tissues or produce false echoes in fluid-filled structures, such as the gallbladder and cysts.

### Time Gain Compensation (TGC)

The power of sound waves is weakened by various factors as they pass through tissues. Echoes returning from deeper tissues are weaker (low amplitude) than those from superficial tissues. By amplifying signals returning from deeper tissues, echoes returning from similar reflectors can be represented with the same shade of gray regardless of their depth. The operator uses the TGC buttons to determine the rate of gain.

### Depth

The depth control changes the depth of the field of view. The number of pixels in the image area is fixed. According to the set field of view, the number of pixels representing each square centimeter of the patient is determined. A higher-resolution image is obtained using the smallest depth of field required to view the structure of interest. A small depth of field should be chosen to evaluate superficial structures and a large depth of field for deep tissues.

### Focus

Ultrasound systems have user-controlled focal zones and provide the best-resolution image at the selected focal depth. The multi-focus option available in many systems allows focusing on a wider area. The disadvantage of using multi-focus is that it reduces the frame rate.

### Dynamic Range

This refers to the interval between strong and weak echoes that can be displayed on the monitor in a given time period. Increasing the dynamic range will result in an image with a wider gray range and lower contrast. If the dynamic range is reduced, the image will have a lower grayscale range and increased contract.

### Zoom

This control is used to enlarge structures of interest in real-time or freeze mode.

### Frame Averaging

Increasing frame averaging can increase subtle textural differences but may cause blurring of the image and decrease the effective frame rate. The frame rate should be lowered when examining high-motion tissues such as the heart.

## Interaction of Sound with Tissue

As sound passes through tissues, various factors cause it to lose energy and therefore decrease in amplitude and intensity, which is called attenuation. The amount of attenuation is determined by the tissue through which it passes, the distance it travels, and the frequency of the sound. Four main processes contribute to the weakening of a sound beam: reflection, refraction, absorption, and scattering. All these factors affect the transmitted sound and echoes returning to the transducer.

### Reflection

Reflection occurs at interfaces between soft tissues of different acoustic impedances. At texture interfaces, some of the sound is reflected and some is transmitted to the texture. The rate of reflection depends on the size of the impedance mismatch and the angle of approach to the interface.

High reflection occurs at soft tissue-air or soft tissue-bone interfaces. Since the amount of transmitted sound is small, deep tissues are shaded. Therefore, it is necessary to use a soft tissue window to view deep tissues and avoid air and bone surfaces.

### Refraction

Refraction is the deviation in the path of sound as it passes through tissue interfaces with different transmission rates. As a result of the deviation that occurs in the sound beam with refraction, misregistration can be seen in echoes.

### Absorption

This refers to the transfer of some of the sound energy to the tissue through which it passes. Absorption causes a heating effect and increases in direct proportion to the frequency of the sound. Therefore, high-frequency transducers are not suitable for the examination of deep tissues.

### Scattering

Scattering occurs at interfaces through which sound passes. At an interface equal to the wavelength of the sound, scattering occurs in many directions. The texture of the ultrasound image often provides such scattering.

### Resolution

Resolution is the ability to distinguish echoes. Contrast resolution refers to the ability of the ultrasound device to show differences between tissues with different properties; temporal resolution is the ability to accurately display changes in anatomy over time; and spatial resolution is the ability to separately view structures that are close to each other.

## Artifacts

### Acoustic Shadowing

If the proportion of beam energy attenuated at a given interface is high, very little sound will be transmitted deeper than the interface, resulting in the inability to receive echoes from tissues deeper than the interface. This creates an acoustic shadow behind the interface. This artifact occurs at soft tissue-gas and soft tissue-bone/calcified tissue (stone-like) interfaces. With this artifact, calcifications in soft tissues and stones in the kidney and gallbladder can be distinguished.

### Acoustic Enhancement

This artifact is caused by fluid-filled structures (such as the bladder, gallbladder, and cysts) attenuating sound much less than solid organs (such as the liver and spleen). Thus, echoes from the areas behind fluid-filled structures are brighter than those from areas behind solid tissues at similar levels. Acoustic enhancement is one of the criteria for identifying cysts. The internal structures of cysts are usually anechoic, but they may contain echoes.

### Edge Shadowing

This occurs deep at the edges of round structures when the velocity of sound passing through the round structure is different from the tissue surrounding the round structure. It is caused by the combination of reflection and refraction at the edge of round structures.

### Reverberation Artifact

This artifact occurs as a result of repeated sound reflections between two interfaces, and it is characterized by multiple representations of the same interface in one image. Echoes are placed on the screen according to the time it takes for them to return to the transducer. If an echo repeatedly echoes between two interfaces, each successive returning echo will be perceived as being received from twice the distance of the previous reflection and placed at twice the distance in the image. An example is the reverberation of subcutaneous tissues in the lumen of a distended bladder. This artifact can be improved by changing the angle of insonation.

### Refraction Artifact

The speed of sound in soft tissues has been accepted as 1.540 m/s, and ultrasound devices have been adjusted accordingly. However, as mentioned previously, there is a difference in the transmission rates of tissues. Accordingly, the sound beam is slower in liquids than in solid tissues. Sound returns later to the transducer from this area. As a result, the structures behind this lesion are mistakenly shown as deeper. For example, in a cystic lesion in the liver, the sound is transmitted more slowly than in the liver, and the part of the diaphragm behind the lesion is shown to be deeper.

### Mirror Image Artifact

This occurs when the sound beam encounters a strongly reflective surface, such as the diaphragm. The primary beam is reflected from such a surface (e.g., the diaphragm), but rather than being directly received by the transducer, it encounters another structure in its path (e.g., a nodular lesion) and is reflected to the highly reflective surface (i.e., the diaphragm). It then returns to the transducer. This results in the reflection of the lesion in the liver on the thorax behind the diaphragm.

### Beam Width/Section Thickness Artifact

This artifact is caused by the incorrect positioning of the focal zone and generated by echoes created by a strong reflector located in an expanded beam beyond the focal zone. It typically presents as false echoes in an anechoic field. False echoes seen in the lumen of anechoic organs, such as the gallbladder and bladder, represent this type of artifact. It may be mistaken for debris in the lumen of the bladder and sludge in the gallbladder. It is possible to avoid this artifact by setting the focal zone to the level of depth of interest and placing the transducer in the center of the object under examination.

## Doppler

If the sound of a moving siren approaches a stationary receiver, the reflected sound waves approach each other, and the wavelength decreases and reaches the receiver at a high frequency. On the contrary, if it moves away, the sound waves move away, the wavelength increases, and low-frequency sound reaches the receiver. This phenomenon is called the Doppler effect or shift. Using the Doppler effect allows determining the direction of the moving reflector.

The amount of frequency difference ($\Delta F$) varies depending on the blood flow velocity ($V0$), the frequency of the sound wave when it leaves the source (Ft), the speed of the sound in the tissue ($c$), and the angle of the sound wave with the long axis of the vessel ($\theta$). All these effects are specified in a single equation (Doppler equation):

$$\Delta F = 2 \times \mathrm{Ft} \times V0 \times \cos\theta \,/\, c$$

In the equation given above, the speed of the sound in the tissue ($c$) is taken as 1.540 m/sec on average as a constant. Since other parameters are also specific, the frequency difference mainly depends on the angle. When the Doppler angle is 90°, the Doppler frequency difference is not detected due to cosine (cos) 90° being equal to zero; therefore, the flow is not coded. Although the highest frequency difference can be obtained if the Doppler angle is 0° (cos 0° = 1), this is not possible for large vessels in practice. In cases where the Doppler angle exceeds 60°, the measured velocity values give results much higher than the actual value due to small changes in the angle and large changes in the cos value of the angle. For all these reasons, it is recommended to examine with an angle of 30–60° between the sound waves and the direction of the flow.

The Doppler technology currently used in ultrasound devices is pulse wave Doppler (PW), in which sound waves are sent in the form of pulses. The Doppler shift, which is the shift in time between the sent and received sound wave, shows the level from which the sound is received. The pulse of a sound wave sent within 1 s is called PRF.

Duplex Doppler images are obtained by combining Doppler information with real-time grayscale imaging. In this system, the sound waves returning to the probe are processed to obtain both the real-time image and the Doppler waveform. The resulting Doppler information is displayed as a graphic using spectral Doppler or as an image using color Doppler or power Doppler.

Color Doppler images provide qualitative information about the flow. Therefore, they are often used not alone but in conjunction with the Doppler spectrum, which offers quantitative information in graphic form. This is known as color-flow duplex Doppler imaging. The phase shift determines the color of the flow, i.e., its direction, and the frequency shift determines the color tone, i.e., flow velocity. Any color can be chosen for the direction of the flow. In a two-color diagram in one corner of the screen, the top color shows the flow approaching the transducer, and the bottom shows the one flowing away.

Power Doppler does not provide direction or velocity information. It shows the amplitude of Doppler signals rather than the frequency shift. Thus, a wider range of Doppler shifts can be detected, facilitating the detection of smaller vessels and lower flows.

## Sonographic Anatomy of the Neck

To interpret radiological findings accurately, first, the anatomy of the section should be well-known. Being familiar with sonographic anatomy will make it easier to identify pathologies. A linear transducer with a frequency of 7.5–12 MHz is preferred in the neck sonographic examination. However, if a large mass is encountered, convex transducers can also be used to ensure penetration and fit the mass into the image.

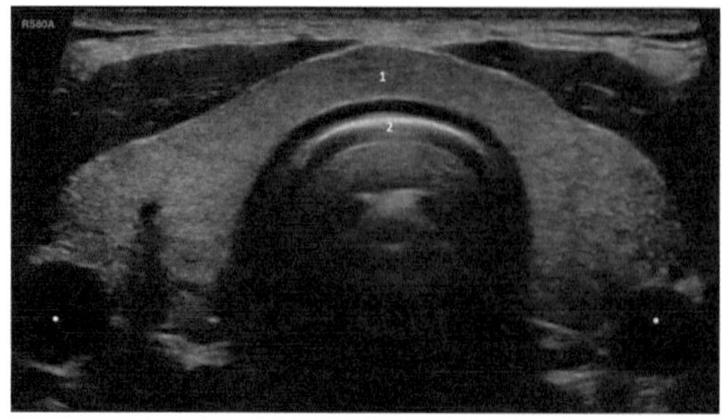

**Fig. 2** Thyroid gland. (1) The thyroid isthmus and (2) the trachea, where the carotid arteries are indicated by (*)

The thyroid gland consists of two lobes and the isthmus connects these lobes. It extends from the level of the fifth cervical vertebra through the level of the first thoracic vertebra. In the infrahyoid plane, the larynx and trachea are located anterolateral to the first ring. The tracheoesophageal groove is located posteromedially, and the carotid space is posterolaterally. The tracheoesophageal groove contains the inferior recurrent nerve, parathyroid glands, and paratracheal lymph nodes. There are infrahyoid strap muscles anteriorly and the sternocleidomastoid muscle anterolaterally. Parathyroid glands are located close to the deep surface of the thyroid gland, and they may sometimes be intracapsular [2, 3].

The thyroid gland has a hyperechoic, homogeneous, intermediate echo concerning the muscles surrounding the gland and presents with a mild internal architecture (Fig. 2). The capsule has a thin hyperechoic appearance [3].

The esophagus is usually located to the left of the trachea, posteromedially to the left lobe of the thyroid (Fig. 3). It consists of a hypoechoic muscle layer that surrounds the echogenic lumen-mucosa-submucosa in the center and the thin echogenic adventitia outside [3, 4].

The parotid gland is the largest salivary gland and is located in the space between the external auditory canal and the inferior mastoid apex and the mandible angle (Fig. 4). There is a superficial

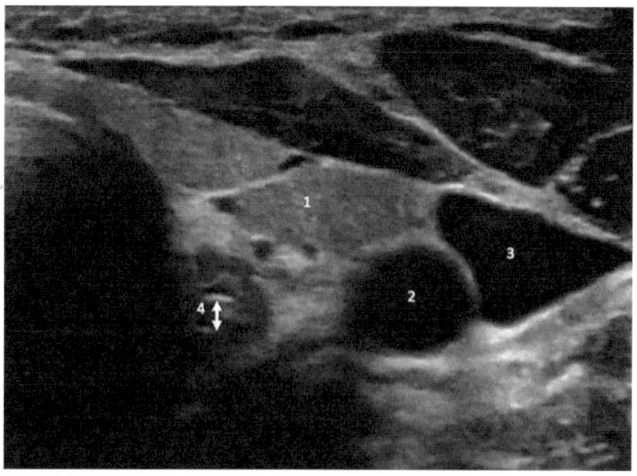


**Fig. 3** Esophagus. (1) The thyroid gland, (2) the carotid artery, (3) the internal jugular vein, and (4) the esophagus (the esophageal lumen is indicated by a double-headed arrow)

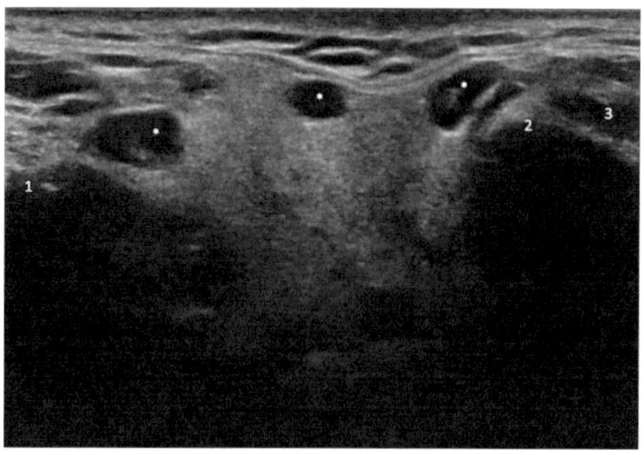


**Fig. 4** Parotid gland. The intraparotid lymph nodes are marked by (*). (1) The mastoid apex, (2) the ramus mandibula, and (3) the masseter muscle

lobe forming 2/3 of the gland and a deep lobe constituting the remaining 1/3. Two vessels are seen just behind the mandibular ramus. The wider laterally located is the retromandibular vein, and the medial is the external carotid artery. The facial nerve lies lateral to the retromandibular vein. After crossing the retromandibular vein, the facial nerve branches off. This crossover demonstrates the surgical distinction between the superficial and deep lobes. The parotid duct emerges from the anterior margin of the gland and, traveling on the surface of the masseter muscle, pierces the buccinator muscle at the level of the second upper molar, opening into the buccal cavity. Along the parotid duct, an accessory parotid gland can be seen on the surface of the masseter muscle [2, 3].

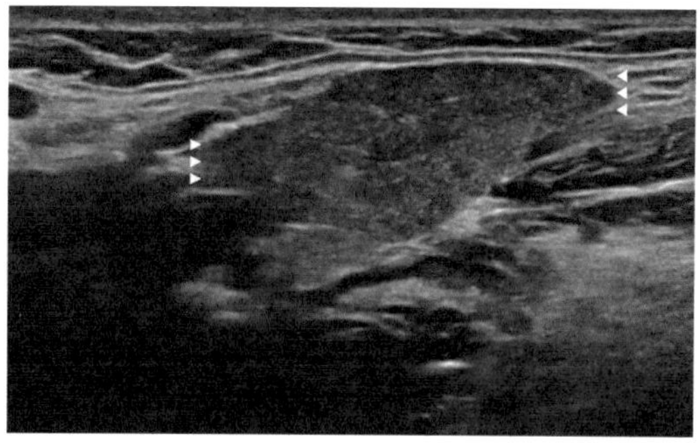

**Fig. 5** Submandibular gland (arrowhead)

The external carotid artery ends 4 cm above the mandible angle, where it divides into the maxillary and temporal arteries. There are approximately 20 intraparotid lymph nodes that do not exceed 5–6 mm in diameter [3]. Fatty infiltration seen with age causes the gland to appear more echogenic and increases the absorption of the sound wave, making it difficult to visualize its deep parts [3, 5, 6]. The facial nerve is indistinguishable from the parotid gland on ultrasound [3, 7].

The submandibular gland is located in the submandibular space (Fig. 5). The submandibular duct emerges from the upper superior surface of the gland and terminates in the last lingual space near the frenulum of the tongue. The gland is uniformly hypoechoic compared to the parotid [5, 6]. Lymph nodes can be seen in the submandibular space, but there are no lymph nodes within the gland.

The sublingual gland lies between the mandible laterally and the floor of the mouth medially. It is located deep, i.e., superior to the mylohyoid muscle. On ultrasound, it is more hyperechoic than the submandibular gland and surrounding muscles [5, 6].

There are carotid spaces on both sides of the neck, where the carotid arteries, internal jugular veins, and cranial nerves are found (cranial nerves 9–12 in the suprahyoid plane and cranial nerve 10 at the infrahyoid level). The common carotid arteries widen at the level of the upper edge of the thyroid cartilage (bifurcation level) and divide into two to form the internal and external carotid arteries (Fig. 6). The common carotid arteries lie posterior to the sternocleidomastoid muscles and medial to the internal

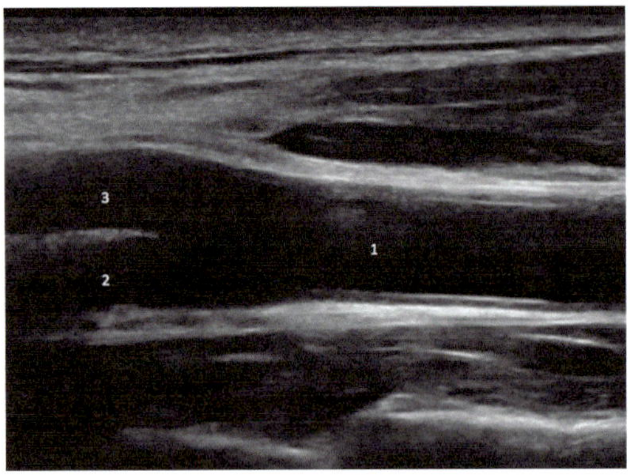


**Fig. 6** Carotid artery. (1) The common carotid artery, (2) the internal carotid artery, and (3) the external carotid artery

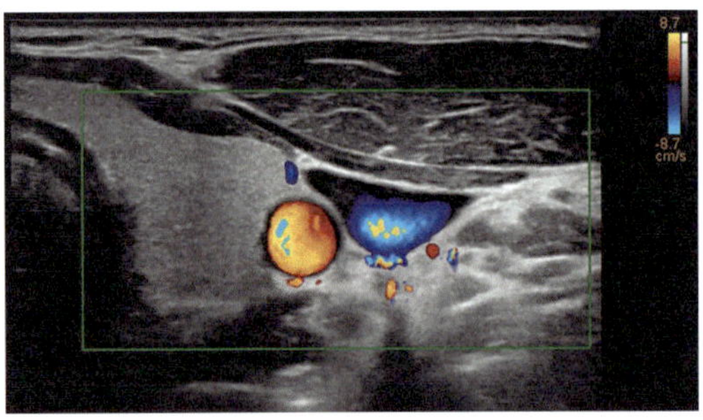


**Fig. 7** The carotid artery and internal jugular vein. The carotid artery is marked using red and the internal jugular vein using blue

jugular veins. The internal jugular veins are posterior to the internal carotid artery and lateral to the common carotid arteries (Fig. 7). The vagus nerve is located at an angle posterior to the common carotid artery and the internal jugular vein [2].

## References

1. Hangiandreou NJ. AAPM/RSNA physics tutorial for residents: topics in US. Radiographics. 2003; 23(4):1019–33.
2. Harnsberger HR, Macdonald AJ. In: Harnsberger HR, Macdonald AJ, editors. Diagnostic and surgical imaging anatomy: brain, head & neck, spine. First. Salt Lake City: Amirsys Inc; 2006.
3. Som PM, Curtin HD. In: Som PM, Curtin HD, editors. Head and neck imaging – 2 volume set: expert consult- online and print. Fifth. St. Louis: Mosby Elsevier; 2011.
4. Ahuja AT, Antonio GE, Wong KT, Wong KT. In: Ahuia AT, Antonio GE, Griffith JF, Ho SY, Wong KT, editors. Diagnostic and surgical imaging anatomy: ultrasound. Salt Lake City: Lippincott Williams & Wilkins; 2007. p. 178–210.
5. Bialek EJ, Jakubowski W, Zajkowski P, Szopinski KT, Osmolski A. US of the major salivary glands: anatomy and spatial relationships, pathologic conditions, and pitfalls. Radiographics. 2006; 26(3):745–63.
6. Gervasio A, D'Orta G, Mujahed I, Biasio A. Sonographic anatomy of the neck: the suprahyoid region. J Ultrasound. 2011;14(3):130–5.
7. Eracleous E, Kallis S, Tziakouri C, Blease S, Gourtsoyiannis N. Sonography, CT, CT sialography, MRI and MRI sialography in investigation of the facial nerve and the differentiation between deep and superficial parotid lesions. Neuroradiology. 1997;39(7):506–11.

## Bibliography

Hangiandreou NJ. AAPM/RSNA physics tutorial for residents: topics in US. Radiographics. 2003;23(4):1019–33.

Boote EJ. AAPM/RSNA physics tutorial for residents: topics in US: doppler US techniques: concepts of blood flow detection and flow dynamics. Radiographics. 2003;23(5):1315–27.

# Cranial Suture Injections for Chronic Migraine

Murat Kara, Yiğit Güngör, and Levent Özçakar

## Introduction

Chronic migraine is a common neurological disorder that affects 1.4–2.2% of the population worldwide [1]. Although the exact underlying pathophysiological mechanism has not been fully/yet understood, the main mechanisms include sensitization of the trigeminocervical complex, whereby neurogenic inflammation is considered to generate pain [2]. Receptors for calcitonin gene-related peptide (CGRP), dopamine, serotonin, glutamate, and substance P play a critical role in the activation of meningeal nociceptors. The sensitized trigeminocervical complex stimulates meningeal sensory nerve endings to release pro-inflammatory peptides, which leads to vasodilation in the dura. As a result, meningeal pain is perceived in extracranial—periorbital, occipital, and temporal—areas through respective somatic afferent nerve fibers, which also innervate homologous areas in the spinal trigeminal nucleus. Especially extracranial meningeal nerve fibers that cross through the cranial sutures are thought to be responsible for temporal or periorbital pain sensation [3, 4].

Treatment of chronic migraine is quite challenging in clinical practice. During the last 10 years, injection of botulinum toxin A (BoNT-A) into the pericranial and neck muscles has been used as an established and approved treatment method. Through this procedure, BoNT-A achieves the blocking of acetylcholine release at motor endplates and nociceptive peptide release (CGRP and the other peptides) from the terminals of C-fiber nociceptors, thereby preventing peripheral sensitization, reducing afferent activity in the C-fibers, and eventually decreasing central sensitization [5]. PREEMPT (Phase III Research Evaluating Migraine Prophylaxis Therapy) studies introduced "31-37 fixed-site and fixed-dose (155-185 U, 5 U/site) intramuscular injections" across head and neck muscles with "follow-the-pain" methodologies [6, 7]. As such, (non-specific) injection sites to the pericranial and neck muscles were not selected according to the abovementioned neurogenic inflammation pathways. In addition, it is difficult to achieve correct localization and depth for blind BoNT injections in the targeted muscles. Moreover, neurogenic inflammation in the dura is postulated to be the essential mechanism in pain generation. Accordingly, injecting BoNT in sutural regions could be safer, more efficient, and/or cost-effective [8–12]. BoNT is quickly absorbed by the nerve endings in the sutural areas, and it then

M. Kara (✉) · L. Özçakar
Hacettepe University Medical School,
Department of Physical and Rehabilitation Medicine,
Ankara, Turkey

Y. Güngör
Kırıkkale University Faculty of Medicine,
Department of Anatomy, Kırıkkale, Turkey



T. Akkaya, A. Cömert (eds.), *Practical Guide for Pain Interventions: Head and Neck Sonoanatomy*,
https://doi.org/10.1007/978-3-031-88773-4_4

reaches meningeal afferent nerve fibers through the orthodromic and antidromic pathways, finally providing pain inhibition. In this regard, it has been shown that BoNT-A can suppress mechanical nociception in peripheral trigeminal neurons in rodents [3]. On the other hand, a novel method of "suture line administration technique using botulinum toxin" has been invented to treat headaches, utilizing patient-specific landmarks [13]. This technique suggested administrating BoNT linearly along at least one suture, but not limited to frontal, squamous, coronal, lambdoidal, occipitomastoid, and sagittal sutures. With this technique, BoNT alleviates the headache within 1–7 days, and its effect lasts about 2–6 months or even longer [13].

Sutural BoNT-A injection extracranially in the sagittal and lambdoid sutures can inhibit nociceptor response to stimulation of the meninges, which was more prominent than when it was injected in the temporalis and neck muscles [11]. Recently, a new injection paradigm (FollowTheSutures) was tested in a pilot study including 20 women with chronic migraine [12]. A total of 90 units of BoNT-A were injected into the 18 perisutural regions by using anatomical landmarks, and patients improved after the injections, with little or no side effects [12]. As precise injection into the sutural areas is crucial, given the high density of afferent nerve collaterals when compared to other cranial areas, it is recommended to apply sutural injections with imaging guidance [8–10]. Accordingly, this chapter discusses BoNT injections into the sutural lines in the cranial area. It requires anatomical information and instructions on ultrasound (US) imaging for cranial sutures. The suggested probe positions and corresponding US images by using a 5–12 MHz linear probe (Logiq P5, GE, Medical Systems, USA) are shown.

## Anatomy and Imaging

The scalp has five layers: skin, subcutaneous tissue (superficial fascia), epicranial muscle and its aponeurosis (galea aponeurotica), subaponeurotic loose areolar tissue, and periosteum of the skull (pericranium) (Fig. 1) [14]. The superficial fascia is firm, dense, fibro-adipose, and closely adherent to the skin and to the underlying muscle and its aponeurosis. The upper layer of the scalp can easily slide on the underlying layer of the loose areolar tissue. Above the zygomatic arch on the upper lateral side of the head, the superficial temporal fascia blends with the galea aponeurotica. A small amount of fat (temporoparietal fat pad) is seen between the superficial fascia and the underlying deep temporal fascia, which continues superiorly as the subgaleal loose areolar tissue in the scalp. The deep temporal fascia is a dense aponeurotic layer that lies under the fat pad and covers the muscle.

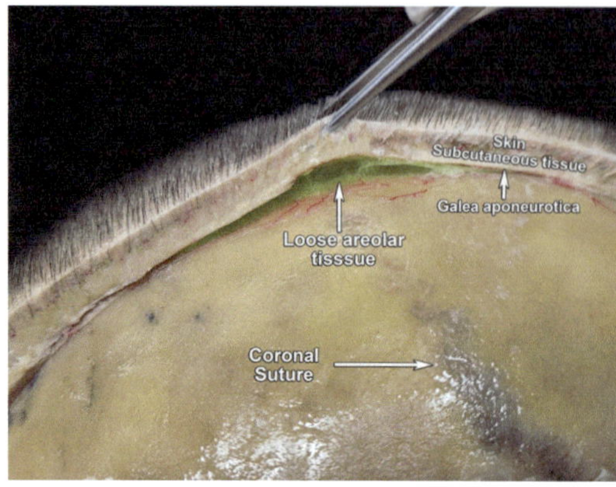


**Fig. 1** Layers of scalp and target area showing skin, subcutaneous tissue (superficial fascia), epicranial muscle and its aponeurosis (galea aponeurotica), subaponeurotic loose areolar tissue, and periosteum of the skull (pericranium)

## Epicranial Muscle (Occipitofrontalis)

Occipitofrontalis covers the dome of the skull from the superior nuchal lines to the eyebrows. It is a wide musculofibrous layer and consists of four thin muscular quadrilateral parts connected by the epicranial aponeurosis. The frontalis muscle is adherent to the superficial fascia, particularly of the eyebrows, and ascends to join the epicranial aponeurosis. Occipitalis arises from the lateral two-thirds of the superior nuchal line of the occiput and the mastoid process of the temporal bone. Occipitalis and frontalis are innervated by the posterior auricular and temporal branches of the facial nerve, respectively. Frontalis raises the eyebrows, and the occipitalis pulls the scalp posteriorly.

## Temporalis Muscle

The temporalis muscle is the largest masticatory muscle. It is fan-shaped and located superficially on the lateral side of the skull. It arises from the temporal fossa up to the inferior temporal line. It attaches to the coronoid process and ramus of the mandible. It is innervated by the mandibular division of the trigeminal nerve. It is divided functionally into a group of vertical fibers that produce mandibular elevation, and more horizontal fibers that produce mandibular elevation and retrusion.

## External Skull and the Sutures

The skull is the most complex bony structure in the body and is composed of 28 separate bones (many of them being paired) [14].The majority of bones articulate with each other by fibrous joints called "sutures". Borders of adjacent bones may be beveled so that the border of one bone overlaps the other (e.g., parietotemporal suture) or may present numerous projections that interlock, giving a serrated jigsaw appearance (e.g. lambdoid suture) [14].

Two parietal bones form most of the cranial roof and sides of the skull. The dentated sagittal part articulates with the opposite parietal bone (*sagittal suture*). The anterior inferior part is overlapped by the greater wing of the sphenoid (*sphenoparietal suture*). The middle inferior part is arched and overlapped by the squamous part of the temporal bone (*squamous suture*). The anterior part is deeply serrated and articulates with the frontal bone (*coronal suture*). The posterior border is deeply dentated and articulates with the occipital bone (*lambdoid suture*). The posterior inferior part is serrated for articulation with the mastoid part (*parietomastoid suture*). Parietomastoid suture meets with the occipitomastoid suture at the lateral end of the lambdoid suture, called "asterion."

## Sagittal Suture

The sagittal suture is a dense and fibrous joint that is located between the two parietal bones (Fig. 1). It lies from the coronal suture in the anterior (*bregma*) to the lambdoid suture in the posterior (*lambda*). The vertex of the skull (the highest point near the middle of the sagittal suture) is palpated on which a high-frequency linear probe is placed coronally to view the suture in the axial view [15]. From that point on, during imaging, the probe is moved backward through serrated contours of the sagittal suture until the L-shaped lambda (the junction between the sagittal and the lambdoid sutures) is viewed. After examining the posterior half of the sagittal suture, the probe is moved forward from the vertex until bregma—a triangular depression where coronal and sagittal sutures meet—is visualized (Fig. 2).

## Squamous Suture

The squamous suture is an arc-shaped suture lying between the parietal bone and the squa-

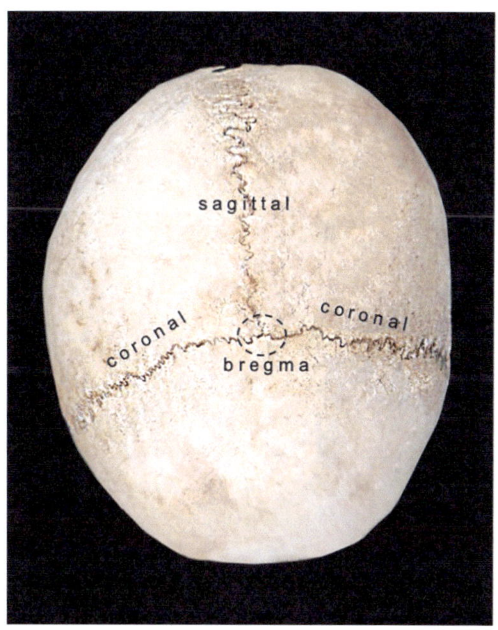


**Fig. 2** The skull view shows the sagittal suture between the two parietal bones and the coronal sutures between the two parietal and the frontal bones

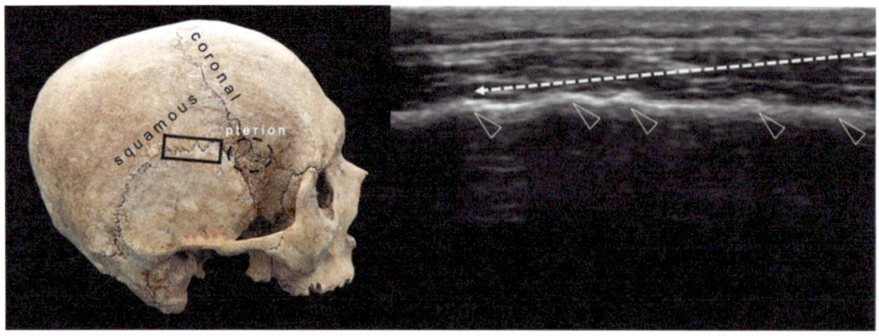


**Fig. 3** The skull view shows the probe position over the squamous suture. The needle (*dashed arrows*) and the cortical irregularity corresponding to the suture can be seen in the long-axis ultrasound view

mous portion of the temporal bone (Fig. 3). The probe is initially placed on the pterion, i.e. the junction of the four bones (frontal, parietal, temporal, and sphenoid bones). Pterion can be palpated as a bony prominence followed by depression when tracking the coronal suture in the inferior direction (Fig. 3). It is an anatomic landmark as it commonly overlies the anterior branch of the middle meningeal artery. The probe can be moved along the natural curve of the squamosal suture in the transverse plane until the parietomastoid suture is scanned. Then, the greater wing of the sphenoid along with sphenofrontal, sphenoparietal, and sphenosquamous sutures can also be visualized.

## Coronal Suture

The coronal suture is a fibrous joint separating the two parietal bones from the frontal bone (Fig. 2). It is located between the right and the left pterions. A high-frequency probe is initially placed on the pterion which is densely occupied by sensory nerve fibers (Fig. 3). It should also be kept in mind that the anterior branch of the meningeal artery lies under the pterion. Afterward, the probe can be moved along the coronal suture passing through the bregma toward the contralateral pterion allowing the coronal suture to be visualized in the sagittal/axial plane.

## Lambdoid Suture

The lambdoid suture is a fibrous joint on the posterior side of the skull separating the parietal bones from the occipital bone (Fig. 4). The lambda is the point where the two parietal bones meet the occipital bone. Accessory sutural bones may be found within a suture (Fig. 5). A large, central interparietal bone can also be seen, called the Inca bone. A high-frequency linear probe is initially placed on lambda which is anticipated as depression and then moved to either side examining the lambdoid suture obliquely in the short-axis until the asterion is viewed [15]. Asterion is an important landmark constituting the junction of parietal, temporal, and occipital bones. Anterior to asterion, the parietomastoid suture can be followed lying between the parietal bone and the mastoid process. Inferomedially, the occipitomastoid suture can be viewed as a depression lying along the posteromedial border of the mastoid process.

## Innervation of the Skull and the Dura Mater

The cranial dura mater is innervated mainly from the three branches of the trigeminal nerve, second and third cervical spinal nerves, and cervical sympathetic trunk [14]. Sensory nerve endings are found only in the dura mater and cerebral blood vessels, not found in the arachnoid pia mater and brain. Additionally, intracranial branches of the trigeminal nerve and high cervical nerves also exit the skull to supply the periosteum and the scalp [14]. The main nerve fibers that pass through the skull—either from the scalp to the dura mater or from the dura mater to the scalp—are unmyelinated C fibers [13]. Interestingly, sensory nerve endings seem to be maximal at the suture lines [13].

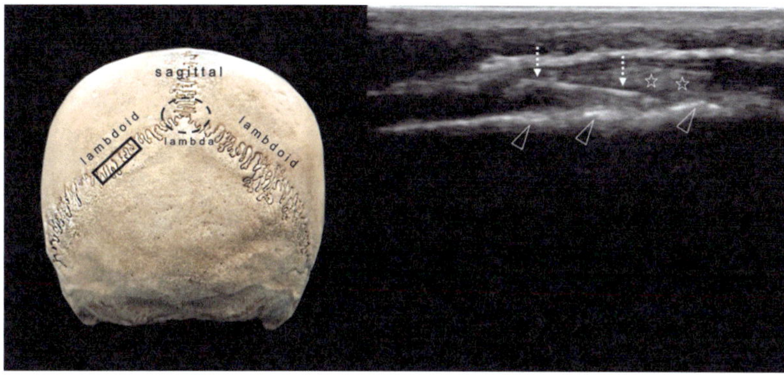


**Fig. 4** The skull view shows the probe positioning during imaging. The corresponding ultrasound image reveals the lambdoid suture (*arrowheads*), the needle (*arrows*), and the toxin (*asterisks*)

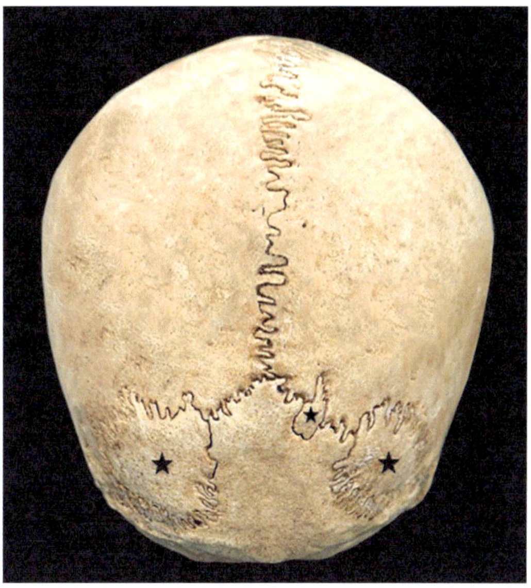

**Fig. 5** The skull view shows the lambdoid suture on the posterior side. Accessory sutural bones (*stars*) may also be found within a suture

## Intervention

After determining the location of the headache, at least one suture line (e.g., squamous, lambdoid, coronal, frontal, and/or sagittal) most proximal to the location can be targeted. The probe can be moved along the natural curve of the cranial suture in the axial plane and then turned in the long-axis view to image the suture line [13]. Thereafter, BoNT-A (or a mixture of corticosteroid and local anesthetic) is continuously administered to the patient along the length of the suture line. It can be injected by utilizing a 27-gauge, 40-mm-length dental needle (or a needle of 1.5 inches in length or 25–30 gauge needles) inserted through the cranial subcutaneous tissue, muscle, and/or aponeurotic fascia along the suture line(s) and then withdrawing the needle gradually while at the same time delivering the toxin [13]. Clinical and sono-palpation findings may be useful in finding the exact injection points for sutures. The direct in-plane method is suggested for the procedure.

## References


1. Kosaras B, Jakubowski M, Kainz V, Burstein R. Sensory innervation of the calvarial bones of the mouse. J Comp Neurol. 2009;515:331–48.
2. Pietrobon D, Striessnig J. Neurobiology of migraine. Nat Rev Neurosci. 2003;4:386–98.
3. Burstein R, Zhang X, Levy D, Aoki KR, Brin MF. Selective inhibition of meningeal nociceptors by botulinum neurotoxin type A: therapeutic implications for migraine and other pains. Cephalalgia. 2014;34:853–69.
4. Schueler M, Messlinger K, Dux M, Neuhuber WL, De Col R. Extracranial projections of meningeal afferents and their impact on meningeal nociception and headache. Pain. 2013;154:1622–31.
5. Becker WJ. Botulinum toxin in the treatment of headache. Toxins (Basel). 2020;12:803.
6. Aurora SK, Dodick DW, Turkel CC, DeGryse RE, Silberstein SD, Lipton RB, et al. PREEMPT 1 Chronic Migraine Study Group Onabotulinum toxin A for treatment of chronic migraine: results from the double-blind, randomized, placebo-controlled phase of the PREEMPT 1 trial. Cephalalgia. 2010;30:793–803.
7. Dodick DW, Turkel CC, DeGryse RE, Aurora SK, Silberstein SD, Lipton RB, et al. PREEMPT Chronic

Migraine Study Group. Onabotulinum toxin A for treatment of chronic migraine: pooled results from the double-blind, randomized, placebo-controlled phases of the PREEMPT clinical program. Headache. 2010;50:921–36.
8. Kara M, Kaymak B, Sekizkardeş M, Özçakar L. The effects/injections of botulinum toxin in chronic migraine headache. Acta Neurol Scand. 2018;138:99.
9. Kara M, Sekizkardeş M, Gürçay E, Akinci A, Özçakar L. Ultrasound-guided perisutural botulinum toxin injection for chronic migraine headache: initial report with technical description. Am J Phys Med Rehabil. 2019;98:e98–e100.
10. Kara M, Gürçay E, Aydın G, et al. Botulinum toxin injections to cranial sutures for chronic migraine. Rewinding the technique using ultrasound imaging. Toxicon. 2019;172:19–22.
11. Zhang X, Strassman AM, Novack V, et al. Extracranial injections of botulinum neurotoxin type A inhibit intracranial meningeal nociceptors' responses to stimulation of TRPV1 and TRPA1 channels: are we getting closer to solving this puzzle? Cephalalgia. 2016;36:875–86.
12. Stovner LJ, Hagen K, Tronvik E, BruvikGravdahl G, Burstein R, Dodick DW. FollowTheSutures: Piloting a new way to administer onabotulinum toxin A for chronic migraine. Cephalalgia. 2022;42(7):590–7. https://doi.org/10.1177/03331024211067775.
13. Standring S. Gray's anatomy: the anatomical basis of clinical practice. 41th ed. Edinburgh: Churchill Livingstone/Elsevier; 2015.
14. Blumenfeld AM. Allergan, Inc., assignee. Suture line administration technique using botulinum toxin. United States patent US 8,617,571 B2; 2013 Dec 31.
15. Kara M, Sekizkardeş M, Akıcıncı A. Peri-sutural injections for migraine. In: Ozcakar L, editor. Ultrasound imaging and guidance for musculoskeletal interventions in physical and rehabilitation medicine. Milan: Edi.Ermes; 2019. p. 31–4.

# Sonoanatomy and Ultrasound Guided Injection for Trigeminal Nerve and Its Branches

Ke-Vin Chang, Wei-Ting Wu, and Levent Özçakar

## Introduction

The lifetime prevalence of trigeminal neuralgia has been reported as 0.3% in a population-based study [1]. A systematic review has highlighted its prevalence to be higher in women than men [2]. Among all the three main branches of the trigeminal nerve, the maxillary and mandibular nerves are mostly involved. Symptom onset is usually aged between 37 and 67 years. The typical symptoms of trigeminal neuralgia include electric shocking or shooting pain over the eyes, jaw, teeth, and gum. The pain is usually unilateral and episodic. Hypertension, excessive dental work, or blow injury to the face are common risk factors for trigeminal neuralgia [3]. The most common origin of trigeminal nerve compression is derived from nearby arteries and veins. The other causes of trigeminal neuralgia include a space-occupying lesion (tumor, cyst, arteriovenous malformation, and bony segment after facial bone fracture) and multiple sclerosis. Other than avoiding the triggers, trigeminal neuralgia management comprises medication (e.g., anticonvulsants) and percutaneous intervention (e.g., injection of local anesthetics and radiofrequency lesioning). Surgery (e.g., microvascular decompression and stereotactic radiosurgery) is reserved for refractory cases [4]. Recently, ultrasound imaging/guidance has been widely used for musculoskeletal injections. Owing to the advances in sonoanatomy of the skull and face [5, 6], ultrasound has already/also been applied for guided injection of the trigeminal nerve. Therefore, this chapter aims to elaborate on the sonoanatomy and ultrasound-guided injection techniques for the trigeminal nerve.

## Superficial Nerve Block

### Supraorbital Nerve

#### Anatomy and Clinical Significance

The supraorbital nerve is a branch of the ophthalmic nerve, i.e., the first branch of the trigeminal

K.-V. Chang (✉)
Department of Physical Medicine and Rehabilitation, National Taiwan University Hospital, Bei-Hu Branch, Taipei, Taiwan

Department of Physical Medicine and Rehabilitation, National Taiwan University College of Medicine, Taipei, Taiwan

Center for Regional Anesthesia and Pain Medicine, Wang-Fang Hospital, Taipei Medical University, Taipei, Taiwan

W.-T. Wu
Department of Physical Medicine and Rehabilitation, National Taiwan University Hospital, Bei-Hu Branch, Taipei, Taiwan

Department of Physical Medicine and Rehabilitation, National Taiwan University College of Medicine, Taipei, Taiwan

L. Özçakar
Hacettepe University Medical School, Department of Physical and Rehabilitation Medicine, Ankara, Turkey



T. Akkaya, A. Cömert (eds.), *Practical Guide for Pain Interventions: Head and Neck Sonoanatomy*,
https://doi.org/10.1007/978-3-031-88773-4_5

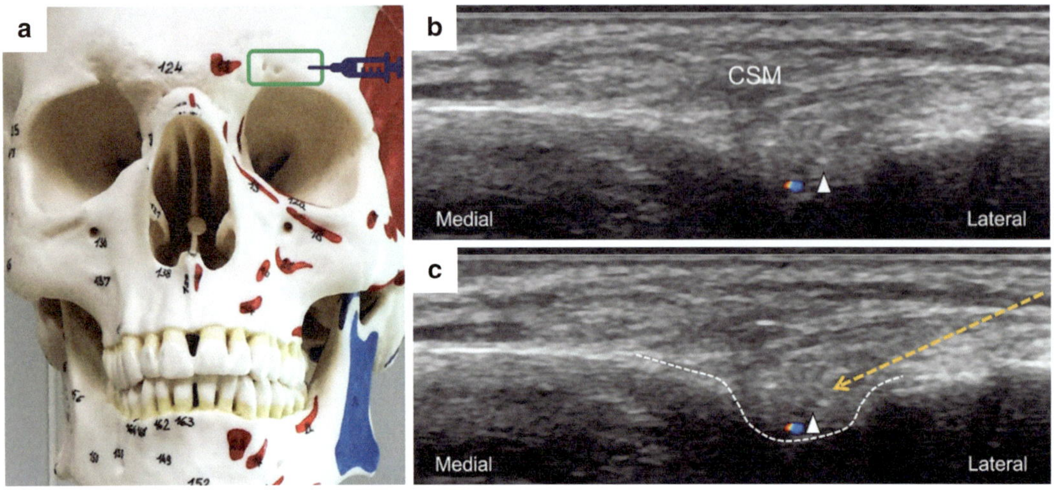


**Fig. 1** Sonoanatomy and ultrasound-guided injection technique for the supraorbital nerve: (**a**) the position of the transducer (green rectangle), (**b**) ultrasound imaging of the supraorbital nerve, (**c**) introducing the needle in lateral-to-medial direction using the in-plane approach to target the supraorbital nerve in the supraorbital notch. The white dashed line denotes the margin of the supraorbital notch. The white arrowhead denotes the supraorbital nerve. The yellow dashed arrow denotes the needle trajectory. CSM corrugator supercilii muscle

nerve (V1). Besides the supraorbital nerve, the ophthalmic nerve also has another branch, i.e., supratrochlear nerve [6, 7]. The supraorbital nerve leaves the skull through the supraorbital notch, a bony aperture at the superior medial aspect of the eye socket. The supraorbital nerve ascends on the forehead, giving off two branches. The medial branch runs over the frontalis muscle, whereas the lateral branch travels over the lateral forehead. In addition to the nerve, the supraorbital notch also harbors the supraorbital artery and vein [5]. The supraorbital nerve is a pure sensory nerve, supplying the skin of the forehead, upper eyelid, and mucosa of the frontal sinus. Patients with neuropathic pain might develop tenderness, hypoesthesia, and allodynia over the innervated region. The compression of the supraorbital nerve can be derived from an orbital fracture, tumor, and helmet or goggles.

### Sonoanatomy and Guided Injection

The transducer is placed in the horizontal plane cranial to the eyebrow whereby the frontalis muscle can be seen along its short axis. Later, the transducer is relocated distally to visualize the orbicularis oculi muscle. The medial end of the transducer is then slightly pivoted toward the bridge of the nose. The supraorbital notch can be found as a discontinuous bony cortex over the supraorbital rim underneath the corrugator supercilii muscle. The supraorbital nerve, along with the cognominal artery and vein, can be identified emerging from the supraorbital notch [8].

When performing the injection, a copious amount of sterilized gel needs to be applied over the lateral end of the transducer. The transducer is then slightly lifted off the skin using the heel-toe maneuver, and the needle is introduced from lateral to medial, using the in-plane approach. The target for injection is the supraorbital notch. Power Doppler imaging should be turned on before the injection to avoid injury to the adjacent vessels (Fig. 1).

## Infraorbital Nerve

### Anatomy and Clinical Significance

The infraorbital nerve branches from the maxillary nerve, i.e., the second branch of the trigeminal nerve (V2) [5, 9]. It leaves the skull through the infraorbital foramen, an orifice located below the eye orbit on the maxillary bone. The nerve is pure sensory and provides innervation to the

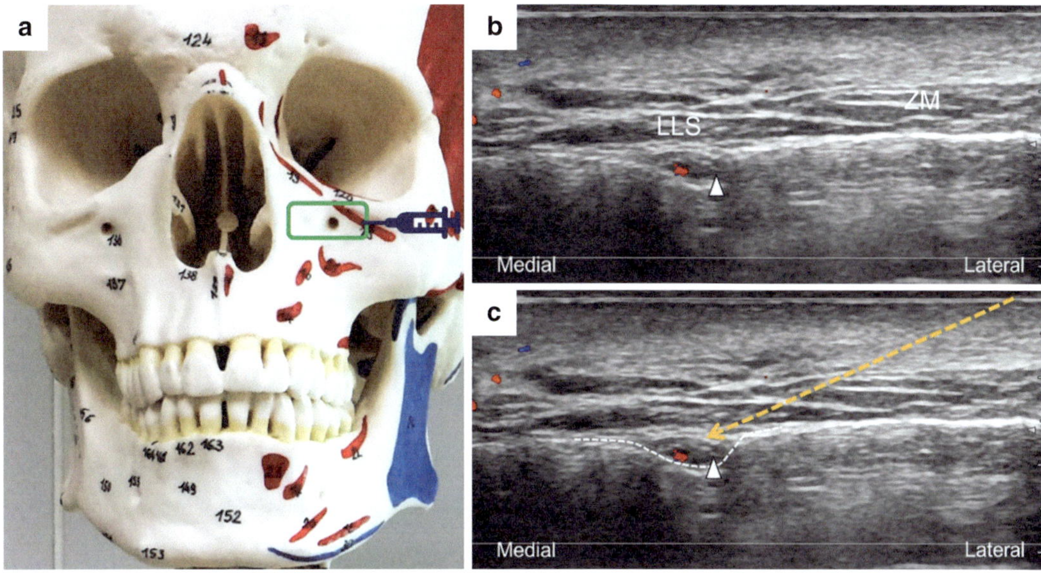


**Fig. 2** Sonoanatomy and ultrasound-guided injection technique for the infraorbital nerve: (**a**) the position of the transducer (green rectangle), (**b**) ultrasound imaging of the infraorbital nerve, (**c**) introducing the needle in lateral-to-medial direction using the in-plane approach to target the infraorbital nerve in the infraorbital foramen. The white dashed line denotes the margin of the infraorbital foramen. The white arrowhead denotes the infraorbital nerve. The yellow dashed arrow denotes the needle trajectory. LLS levator labii superioris muscle, ZM zygomaticus minor muscle

majority of the cheek, ala of the nose and upper lip. The infraorbital artery and vein accompany the nerve, emerging from the infraorbital foramen. Besides the treatment for neuralgia over the area innervated by the infraorbital nerve, other indications comprise wound suture and dental procedures over the relevant regions.

### Sonoanatomy and Guided Injection

The transducer is placed over the middle of the infraorbital rim in the horizontal plane and is then relocated slightly toward the upper lip. The infraorbital foramen can be identified as a concave pit over the maxillary bone, on top of which are the levator labii superioris and levator anguli oris muscles. The infraorbital nerve can be visualized emerging from the infraorbital foramen [8].

During the injection, a copious amount of sterilized gel can be addressed over the lateral end of the transducer, which needs to be lifted off from the underlying skin. The needle is then inserted via lateral-to-medial direction to target the infraorbital foramen. Power Doppler imaging should be turned on to locate the accompanying infraorbital vessels before the injection (Fig. 2).

## Mental Nerve

### Anatomy and Clinical Significance

The mental nerve is the branch of the mandibular nerve, i.e., the third branch of the trigeminal nerve [6, 10]. The nerve exits the skull through the mental foramen, a bilateral opening at the body of the mandible. It is also purely sensory, innervating the anterior portion of the buccal mucosa, lower lip, and anterior chin. In addition to neuralgia over the region supplied by the mental nerve, its blockage can be performed for dermatological procedures over the chin. Of note, as the mental nerve does not provide sensation to the teeth, a mental nerve block would have a limited value in dental procedures of the lower jaw.

### Sonoanatomy and Guided Injection

The transducer is placed in the horizontal plane inferior to the lower lip. It is then relocated

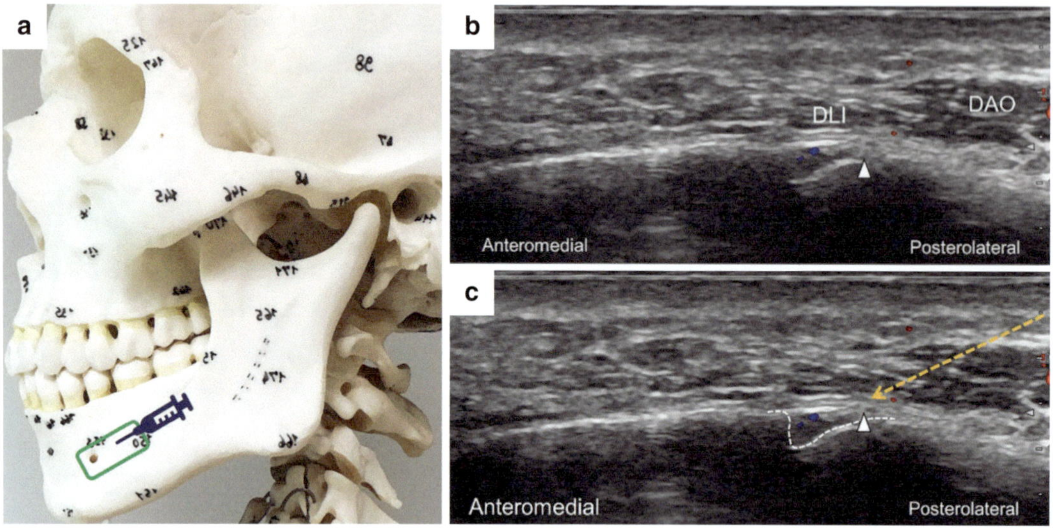


**Fig. 3** Sonoanatomy and ultrasound-guided injection technique for the mental nerve: (**a**) the position of the transducer (green rectangle), (**b**) ultrasound imaging of the mental nerve, (**c**) introducing the needle in the posterolateral-to-anteromedial direction using the in-plane approach to target the mental nerve in the mental foramen. The white dashed line denotes the mental foramen. The white arrowhead denotes the mental nerve. The yellow dashed arrow denotes the needle trajectory. DLI depressor labii inferioris muscle, DAO depressor anguli oris muscle

upward or downward to locate the mental foreman. The mental nerve can be visualized emerging from the mental foramen underneath the mentalis, depressor labii inferioris, and depressor anguli oris muscles [8].

When performing the injection, a copious amount of sterilized gel can be placed between one edge of the transducer, with the same end lifted off against the skin. The needle is inserted from the lateral end of the transducer, targeting the mental foramen. Prior to the injection, the power Doppler mode should be turned on to avoid accidental injury to the inferior labial artery (Fig. 3).

## Deep Nerve Block

### Maxillary Nerve

#### Anatomy and Clinical Significance

The maxillary nerve is the second division of the trigeminal nerve and is rooted from the semilunar ganglion [11]. It exits the skull base through the foramen rotundum and enters the pterygopalatine fossa, a cone-shaped depression deep to the infratemporal fossa. The maxillary nerve passes through the pterygopalatine ganglion and carries the post-ganglionic sympathetic and parasympathetic fibers to the terminal branches, including zygomatic, (posterior, middle, and anterior) superior alveolar, pharyngeal, infraorbital, and superior labial nerves. The maxillary nerve can be involved by trauma, tumors, aneurysms, and infection. In patients with trigeminal neuralgia over the V2 division, magnetic resonance imaging or computed tomography should be arranged for scrutinizing the aforementioned pathologies.

#### Sonoanatomy and Guided Injection

The curvilinear transducer is placed in the horizontal plane over the zygomatic arch and is then relocated distally [8, 12]. The masseter, temporalis, and lateral pterygoid muscles can be seen in a superficial-to-deep arrangement. Asking the patient to slightly open the mouth can be helpful to enlarge the window between the zygomatic arch and condylar process of the mandible. The most important landmark is the lateral pterygoid plate, where the lateral pterygoid muscle attaches to. The lateral pterygoid muscle is triangular-shaped, whereby its origin can be identified on

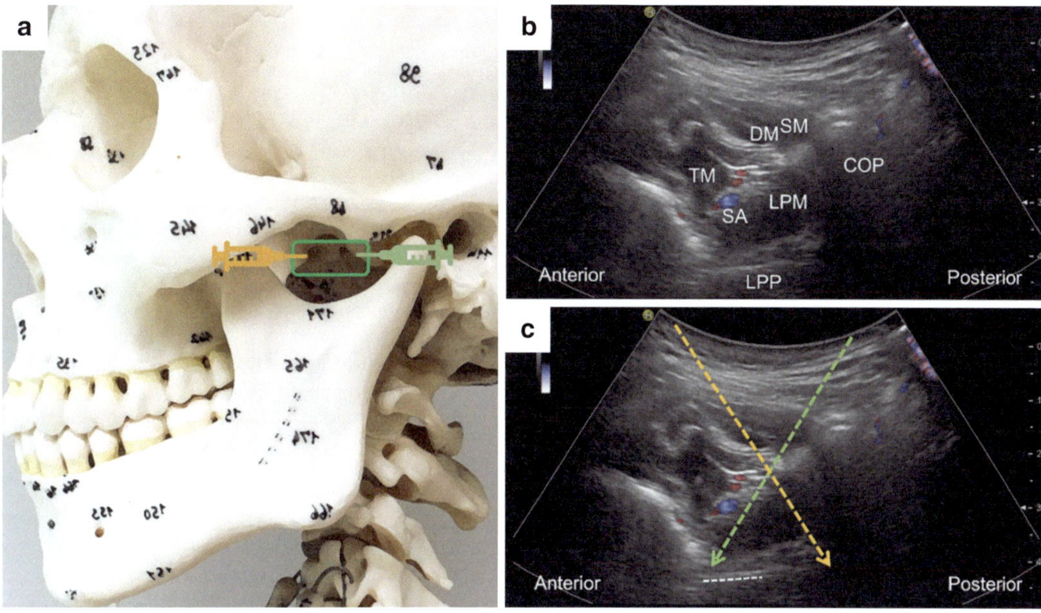


**Fig. 4** Sonoanatomy and ultrasound-guided injection technique for the maxillary and mandibular nerves: (**a**) the position of the transducer (green rectangle), (**b**) color Doppler image during mouth opening, and (**c**) introducing the needle using the in-plane approach to target the nerves. The green dashed arrow represents the needle trajectory for injection of the maxillary nerve, while the yellow dashed arrow represents the needle trajectory for injection of the mandibular nerve. The white dash denotes the lateral pterygoid plate. COP condylar process, DM deep masseter, SM superficial masseter, LPM lateral pterygoid muscle, LPP lateral pterygoid plate, TM temporalis muscle, SA sphenopalatine artery

the condylar process of the mandible. During the injection, the needle is introduced through out-of-plane approach, targeting the pterygopalatine fossa anterior to the lateral pterygoid plate. The sphenopalatine artery, a branch of the maxillary artery, should be checked before injection using the power Doppler mode. As the maxillary nerve cannot be really identified under ultrasound, concomitant use of electrostimulation and fluoroscopy would facilitate the precise location of the nerve (Fig. 4).

## Mandibular Nerve

### Anatomy and Clinical Significance

Mandibular nerve is the third division of trigeminal nerve and also stems from the semilunar ganglion [8, 13]. It is the only branch carrying fibers from the motor root of the trigeminal nerve. The mandibular nerve exits the skull through the foramen ovale and arrives at the infratemporal fossa. In the intracranial region, the mandibular nerve sends the sensory meningeal branch and motor branches to innervate the medial pterygoid, tensor tympani, and tensor veli palatini muscles. In the extracranial region, the mandibular nerve provides motor innervation to the temporalis, masseter, lateral pterygoid, mylohyoid, and anterior belly of digastric muscles. Its sensory contribution includes the mandibular teeth, chin, lower lip, and ear (via the auriculotemporal nerve). The territory innervated by the mandibular nerve is a common place for trigeminal neuralgia. Mandibular nerve block can be performed for analgesia during dental procedures of the lower jaw or for pain due to temporomandibular joint disorders.

### Sonoanatomy and Guided Injection

The transducer placement is similar to the maxillary nerve injection described above [8]. The curvilinear transducer is placed in the horizontal plane over the zygomatic arch and is then relocated distally. The patient is asked to slightly open the mouth to enlarge the window between the zygomatic arch and condylar process of the mandible. The needle is introduced through the inferior edge of the transducer using the out-of-plane approach, targeting the region posterior to the lateral pterygoid plate (Fig. 4). The needle tip should be directed toward the infratemporal fossa. Before injection, the power Doppler mode must be turned on to avoid injury to the maxillary artery. Likewise, the mandibular nerve cannot be directly visualized under ultrasound imaging, and concomitant use of electrostimulation and fluoroscopy would be helpful for localizing the nerve precisely.

## Conclusion

Ultrasound imaging is helpful to identify the bony landmarks essential while blocking the trigeminal nerve branches. Prior to the injection, the power Doppler mode should be turned on to confirm the location of adjacent vessels. During the deep blockage of the trigeminal nerve, electrostimulation and fluoroscopy would be of additional help to ultrasound guidance for determining the best/optimal injection site.

## References

1. Mueller D, Obermann M, Yoon M-S, et al. Prevalence of trigeminal neuralgia and persistent idiopathic facial pain: a population-based study. Cephalalgia. 2011;31(15):1542–8.
2. De Toledo IP, Conti Réus J, Fernandes M, et al. Prevalence of trigeminal neuralgia: a systematic review. J Am Dent Assoc. 2016;147(7):570–6.e2.
3. Duransoy YK, Mete M, Akçay E, Selçuki M. Differences in individual susceptibility affect the development of trigeminal neuralgia. Neural Regen Res. 2013;8(14):1337–42.
4. Xu R, Xie ME, Jackson CM. Trigeminal neuralgia: current approaches and emerging interventions. J Pain Res. 2021;14:3437–63.
5. Wu WT, Chang KV, Chang HC, et al. Ultrasound imaging of facial vascular neural structures and relevance to aesthetic injections: a pictorial essay. Diagnostics (Basel). 2022;12(7):1766.
6. Wu WT, Chang KV, Chang HC, et al. Ultrasound imaging of the facial muscles and relevance with botulinum toxin injections: a pictorial essay and narrative review. Toxins (Basel). 2022;14(2):101.
7. Napier A, De Jesus O, Taylor A. Supraorbital nerve block. In: StatPearls. Treasure Island: StatPearls Publishing. Copyright © 2022, StatPearls Publishing LLC.; 2022.
8. Allam AE, Khalil AAF, Eltawab BA, Wu WT, Chang KV. Ultrasound-guided intervention for treatment of trigeminal neuralgia: an updated review of anatomy and techniques. Pain Res Manag. 2018;2018:5480728.
9. Nardi NM, Alvarado AC, Schaefer TJ. Infraorbital nerve block. In: StatPearls. Treasure Island: StatPearls Publishing. Copyright © 2022, StatPearls Publishing LLC.; 2022.
10. Betz D, Fane K. Mental nerve block. In: StatPearls. Treasure Island: StatPearls Publishing. Copyright © 2022, StatPearls Publishing LLC.; 2022.
11. Shafique S, Das JM. Anatomy, head and neck, maxillary nerve. In: StatPearls. Treasure Island: StatPearls Publishing. Copyright © 2022, StatPearls Publishing LLC.; 2022.
12. Chang KV, Lin CS, Lin CP, Wu WT, Ozcakar L. Recognition of the lateral pterygoid muscle and plate during ultrasound-guided trigeminal nerve block. J Clin Diagn Res. 2017;11(5):UL01–UL2.
13. Ghatak RN, Helwany M, Ginglen JG. Anatomy, head and neck, mandibular nerve. In: StatPearls. Treasure Island: StatPearls Publishing. Copyright © 2022, StatPearls Publishing LLC.; 2022.

# Other Facial Procedures (Supraorbital, Infraorbital, and Mental Nerve Blocks)

Halil Cetingok, Gül Koknel Talu, and Ozcan Gayretli

## Introduction

Many pain syndromes are present in the face, such as trigeminal neuralgia, postherpetic neuralgia, atypical facial neuralgia, migraine, pain related to the temporomandibular joint or teeth, etc. Pain impulses originating from nociceptors in the face area are transmitted by the trigeminal nerve (fifth cranial nerve: CN V) and its branches [1]. The sensory ganglion of the trigeminal nerve is the gasserian (semilunar) ganglion, and it is located in the Meckel cave at the apex of the petrous portion of the temporal bone in the middle cranial fossa [1].

Three major divisions arise from the Gasserian ganglion: ophthalmic (V1), maxillary (V2), and mandibular (V3). These main divisions provide sensory innervation of deep and superficial structures in the face region by dividing into terminal branches. Among them, the supraorbital branch of the ophthalmic division, the infraorbital branch of the maxillary division, and the mental branch of the mandibular division are the main neural structures that compose the skin and subcutaneous sense of the facial region by ascending to the cutaneous area through the relevant foramen (Figs. 1 and 2) [2]. In cases of allodynia, hyperalgesia, and triggering by stimulus in the neuropathic pain syndromes, these nerves show nociceptive activity in related dermatomes. Therefore, there are many diagnostic and therapeutic procedures since the blockade of these nerves prevents pain transmission.

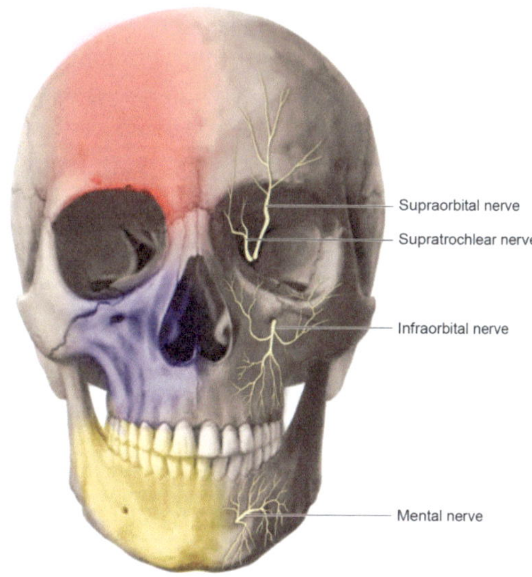


**Fig. 1** Supraorbital, infraorbital, mental nerves, and relevant dermatome. *nerve distribution on one side and related cutaneous dermatomal area on the other

H. Cetingok (✉) · G. K. Talu
Istanbul University, Istanbul Faculty of Medicine, Department of Anesthesiology, Division of Pain Medicine, İstanbul, Türkiye
e-mail: halil.cetingok@istanbul.edu.tr; gul.talu@istanbul.edu.tr

O. Gayretli
Istanbul University, Istanbul Faculty of Medicine, Department of Anatomy, İstanbul, Türkiye
e-mail: gayretli@istanbul.edu.tr



T. Akkaya, A. Cömert (eds.), *Practical Guide for Pain Interventions: Head and Neck Sonoanatomy*,
https://doi.org/10.1007/978-3-031-88773-4_6

In routine clinical practice, these nerves are blocked by palpation of the foramen in possible locations with landmark methods. But, in some cases, it is difficult to determine the exact localization of the nerve, and the vascular structures adjacent to the nerve may be damaged during the block. In addition, considering the possible anatomic variations such as double foramen, accessory nerve, and aberrant vascular structure, it is accepted that the use of imaging techniques is beneficial [3]. Ultrasound, which can visualize soft tissues in real time, can show the relevant foramens, and the neural and vascular structures arising from them [3]. It is also important to be able to advance the needle enough to block the nerve while staying away from structures that may cause complications. Also, to see the spread of the injected solution with ultrasound guidance is very important. As a consequence, concerning developments in techniques and technology, radiologic guidance is a"must" for blocking the nerve.

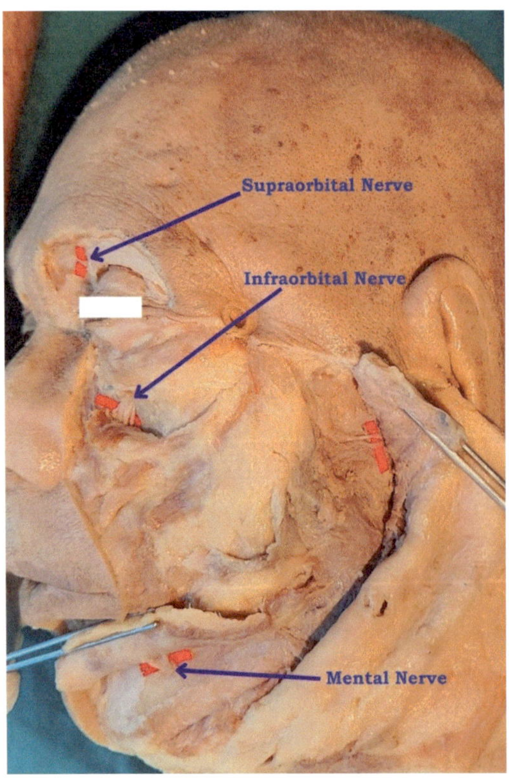


**Fig. 2** Supraorbital, infraorbital, mental nerves in cadaver

In this chapter, the anatomy of the cutaneous terminal branches of the trigeminal nerve, its sonoanatomy, ultrasound-guided blockade techniques, indications, and complications are explained.

## Supraorbital Nerve Block

### Supraorbital Nerve Anatomy

The supraorbital nerve is one of the terminal branches of the ophthalmic division (CN V1) of the trigeminal nerve and provides ipsilateral sensory innervation to the forehead, upper eyelid, and anterior scalp to the vertex of the skull (Fig. 3) [4].

The ophthalmic nerve exits the skull and enters the orbit via the superior orbital fissure and divides into the lacrimal nerve, the nasociliary nerve, and the frontal nerve [1]. The frontal nerve is the largest branch of the ophthalmic nerve and gives terminal branches: the supraorbital nerve (larger lateral) and the supratrochlear nerve (smaller medial) [1]. The supraorbital nerve exits the orbit via the supraorbital notch or foramen with supraorbital arteries, then runs up to the forehead, passing through the corrugator muscle and dividing into medial and lateral branches [5].

The supraorbital notch/foramen lies on the frontal bone, and it is approximately 20–25 mm lateral to the midline (Fig. 4) [6]. The supraorbital nerve passes through a notch (83%) or a bony foramen (27%) [7]. Supraorbital notch has approximately 7–8 mm depth, and it is usually covered by a fascial band (86%) [7].

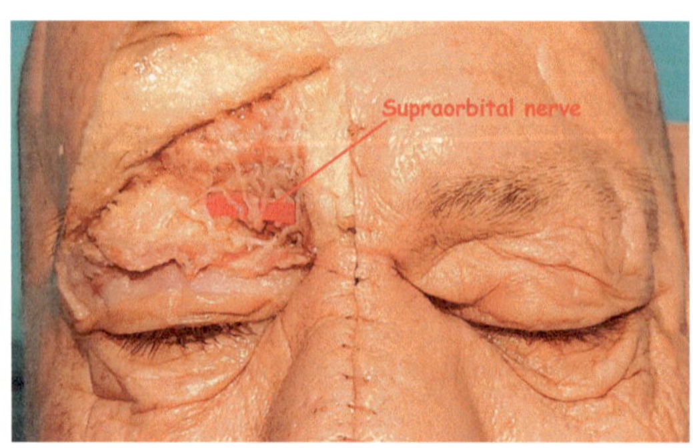


**Fig. 3** Supraorbital nerve in cadaver

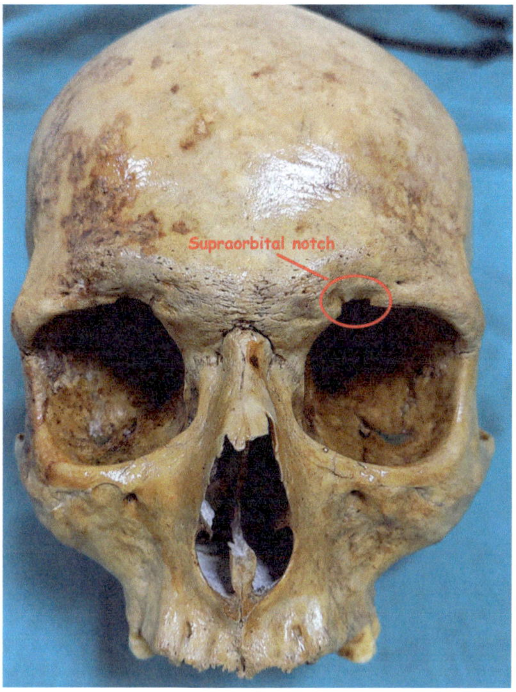


**Fig. 4** Supraorbital notch/foramen in the skull

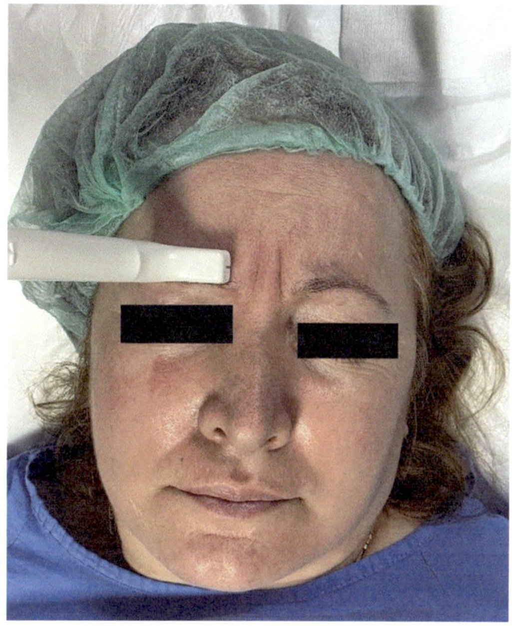

**Fig. 5** Probe placement in ultrasound-guided supraorbital nerve block

## Ultrasound-Guided Supraorbital Nerve Block

### Indications

Supraorbital nerve block is useful in the diagnosis and treatment of painful conditions in areas innervated by the supraorbital nerve [4, 5, 8, 9]:

- Trigeminal neuralgia and neuropathy (V1 distribution)
- Acute herpes zoster and post-herpetic neuralgia (V1 distribution)
- Supraorbital neuralgia and nerve entrapment
  - Trauma/fractures of the orbital roof
  - Tumors of the orbit
  - Tight swimming goggles or motorcycle helmet
  - Foraminal stenosis due to Paget's disease
- Diagnosis of trigger points and hyperalgesic zones in the supraorbital region
- Providing surgical anesthesia or postoperative analgesia in the innervation area of the supraorbital nerve

### Ultrasound-Guided Technique

The patient is placed in the supine position. The supraorbital notch/foramen is identified by palpation with the index finger at the upper edge of the orbit (approximately 2.5 cm lateral to midline or at the mid-pupillary line) [6, 10]. The skin covering the notch/foramen is cleaned with an antiseptic solution and prepped in a sterile fashion. On ultrasound, the bone structures are typically shown as hyperechoic (bright) linear lines and the deep tissue behind them as hypoechoic (dark) [11]. A high-frequency linear or hockey stick transducer is placed along the supraorbital notch/foramen in a transverse plane, and the bone structure is seen as a linear line just 5–10 mm below the surface (Fig. 5). The supraorbital notch is visualized as a bony defect or discontinuity on the hyperechoic supraorbital ridge [12, 13]. Then the supraorbital nerve and artery (using color Doppler mode) are identified in the notch. The 25–27-gauge, 5 cm blunt-tipped nerve block needle is placed toward the supraorbital notch/foramen in-plane technique, lateral to the medial direction (Fig. 6). After touching the bone, the tip is slightly withdrawn. Following negative aspira-

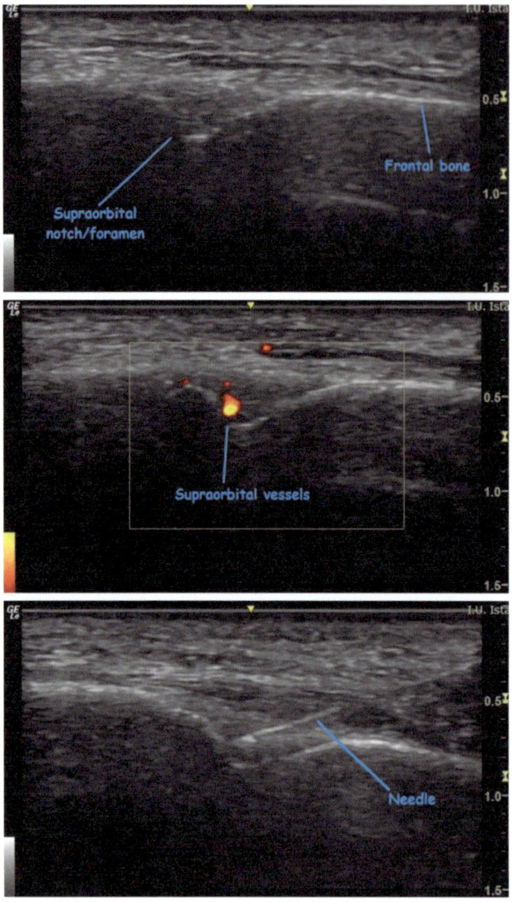


**Fig. 6** Ultrasound-guided supraorbital nerve block

tion, 2–3 ml of local anesthetic solution (bupivacaine 0.5% or lidocaine 2% with or without corticosteroid) is injected. In order not to cause mechanical damage to the supraorbital nerve with the tip of the needle or compressive damage to the supraorbital nerve with the injectate, placement of the tip of the needle in the foramen should be avoided [8, 14]. During the injection, the gauze sponge should be applied with gentle pressure on the upper eyelid to prevent the spread of the solution to the soft tissue of the upper eyelid [4]. After the block procedure, pressure should be applied to the injection site to prevent bleeding and hematoma formation [8].

The blockade provides anesthesia in the dermatome area of the nerve. It allows for a diagnosis to determine whether the supraorbital nerve is present in the pain pathway. Or therapeutically, it provides analgesia in the relevant area. Mostly the resulting analgesia is short-lived and ends when the effect of the local anesthetic solution on the nerve disappears. However, longer-lasting effects can be obtained by methods such as adding steroids to the solution, making repetitive blocks, using thermal radiofrequency ablation, cryoablation, or chemical neurolysis [5].

### Complications [5, 8, 10, 15]

- Bleeding and hematoma (if adequate compression is not provided)
- Swelling, redness, ecchymosis on the skin
- Alopecia and skin atrophy (steroid use and its subcutaneous spread)
- Compression neuropathy (inserting the needle into the foramen and injecting)
- Neuritis (especially for neurolytic injections)
- Infection (rare)
- Allergic reaction to the injectate
- Temporary ptosis (effect of local anesthetics on levator palpebrae muscle)
- Cardiac arrhythmias (due to oculocardiac reflex via the trigeminal nerve)

## Infraorbital Nerve Block

### Infraorbital Nerve Anatomy

The infraorbital nerve is the terminal branch of the maxillary division (CN V2) of the trigeminal nerve and provides ipsilateral sensory innervation to the lower eyelid, lateral nares, upper lip, upper teeth, and associated gingiva (Fig. 7) [4].

The maxillary nerve is solely sensory [1]. It exits the skull via the foramen rotundum and enters the sphenopalatine (pterygopalatine) fossa [1]. Then it enters the orbit through the inferior orbital fissure and courses along the floor of the orbit in the infraorbital groove [1, 16]. The maxillary nerve's main root becomes the infraorbital nerve and exits the orbit through the infraorbital foramen with infraorbital arteries [1, 16]. After ascending to the maxillary region, it proceeds deep into the levator labii superioris muscle [12].

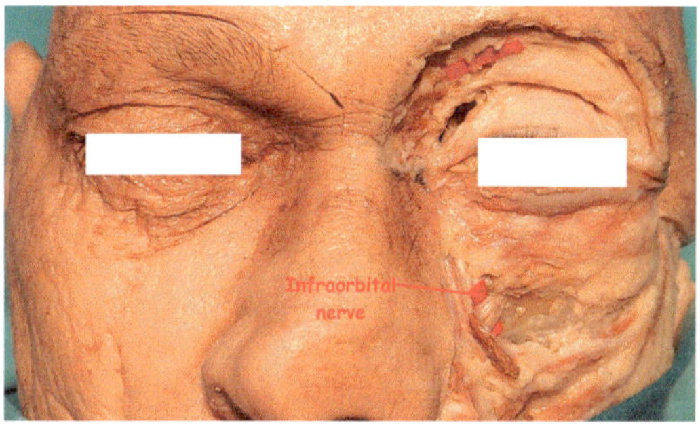


**Fig. 7** Infraorbital nerve in cadaver

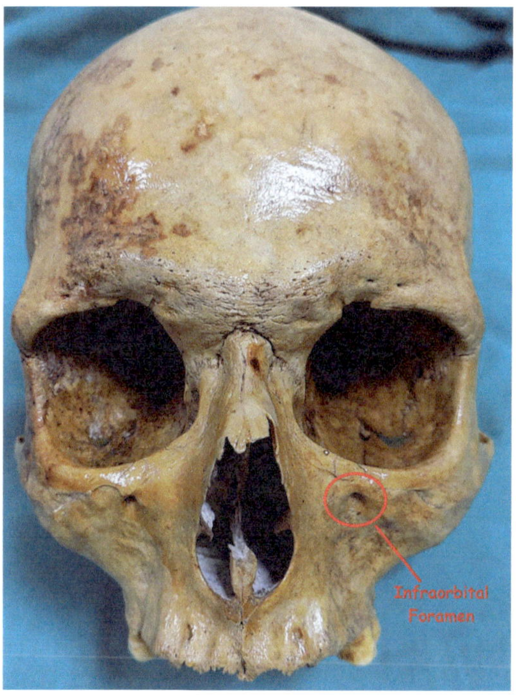


**Fig. 8** Infraorbital foramen in skull

The infraorbital foramen lies on the maxilla bone, and it is approximately 5–8.5 mm below the inferior orbital rim and 20–25 mm lateral to the midline (nearly in the same vertical line with the supraorbital notch) (Fig. 8) [17]. The most common shape of the infraorbital foramen is oval. Approximately, 21% of cases have accessory infraorbital foramens, mostly on one side and superomedial to the infraorbital foramen [17].

## Ultrasound-Guided Infraorbital Nerve Block

### Indications

Infraorbital nerve block is useful in the diagnosis and treatment of painful conditions in areas sensed by the infraorbital nerve [4, 8, 9, 16]:

- Trigeminal neuralgia and neuropathy (V2 distribution)
- Acute herpes zoster and post-herpetic neuralgia (V2 distribution)
- Infraorbital neuralgia and nerve entrapment
  - Trauma/fractures of the zygoma
  - Tumors of the maxilla
  - Maxillary sinusitis
  - Foraminal stenosis due to Paget's disease
- Diagnosis of trigger points and hyperalgesic zones in the infraorbital region
- Providing surgical anesthesia or postoperative analgesia in the innervation area of the infraorbital nerve

### Ultrasound-Guided Technique

The patient is placed in the supine position. The infraorbital foramen is identified by palpation with the index finger at the maxilla (approximately, 5–8.5 mm below the inferior orbital rim, 2.5 cm lateral to midline or at the mid-pupillary line) [17]. The skin covering the foramen is cleaned with an antiseptic solution and prepped in a sterile fashion. On ultrasound, the bone structure is typically shown as hyperechoic (bright) linear lines, and the deep tissue behind them as hypoechoic (dark) [11]. A high-frequency linear or hockey stick transducer is placed along the infraorbital foramen in a longitudinal plane (Fig. 9). The infraorbital foramen is visualized as a bony defect or discontinuity on the hyperechoic maxilla [14]. The area should be scanned by placing the probe in the longitudinal plane and sliding it medially and laterally. While the foramen is detected as a defective appearance in the maxilla, it is seen that the bone structure in the maxilla is uninterrupted when the probe is shifted more medially or laterally. On the other hand, approxi-

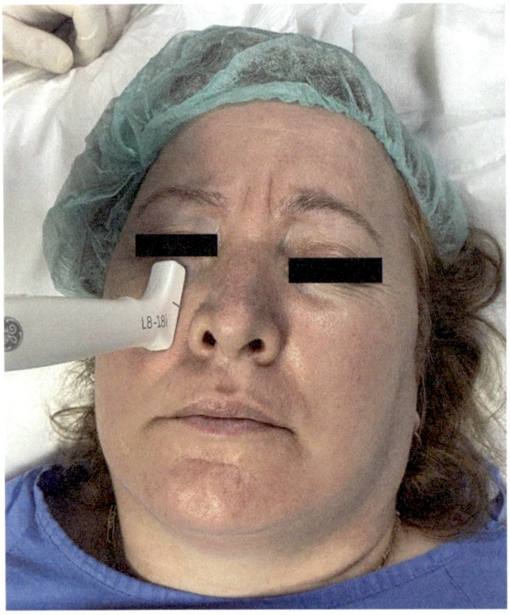


**Fig. 9** Probe placement in ultrasound-guided infraorbital nerve block

mately 18% of patients have an accessory infraorbital foramen and nerve (usually superolaterally located) [18]. In order not to miss the accessory foramen or to avoid accidentally blocking only the accessory foramen and nerve, the area should be scanned with the ultrasound probe. Then the infraorbital nerve and artery (using color Doppler mode) are identified in the notch. The 25–27-gauge, 5 cm blunt-tipped nerve block needle is placed toward the infraorbital foramen in the in-plane technique, caudocranial direction (Fig. 10). After touching the bone, the tip is slightly withdrawn. Following negative aspiration, 2–3 ml of local anesthetic solution (bupivacaine 0.5% or lidocaine 2% with or without corticosteroid) is injected. In order not to cause mechanical damage to the infraorbital nerve with the tip of the needle or compressive damage to the infraorbital nerve with the injectate, placement of the tip of the needle in the foramen should be avoided [8, 10, 14]. Another important point to note is that it is necessary to avoid accidentally injecting into the orbit [10, 18]. After the block procedure, pressure should be applied to the injection site to prevent bleeding and hematoma formation [8].

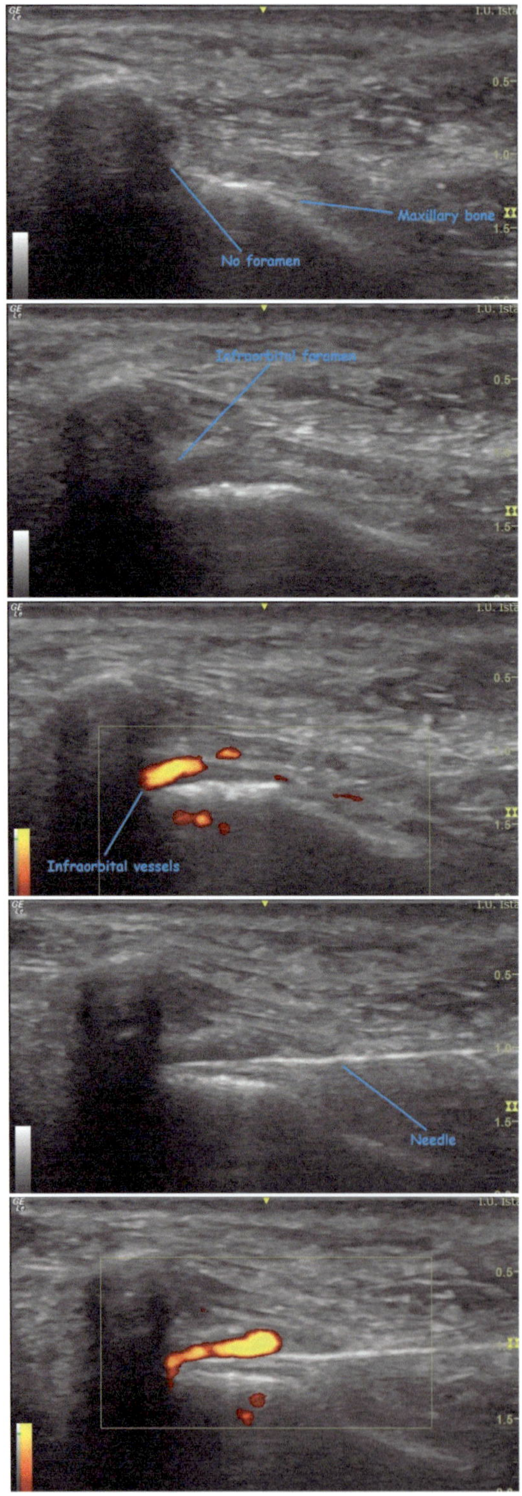


**Fig. 10** Ultrasound-guided infraorbital nerve block

The blockade provides anesthesia in the dermatome area of the nerve. It allows diagnostically to determine whether the supraorbital nerve is present in the pain pathway. Or therapeutically, it provides analgesia in the relevant area. Mostly the resulting analgesia is short-lived and ends when the effect of the local anesthetic solution on the nerve disappears. However, longer-lasting effects can be obtained by methods such as adding steroids to the solution, making repetitive blocks, using thermal radiofrequency ablation, cryoablation, or chemical neurolysis [16, 19].

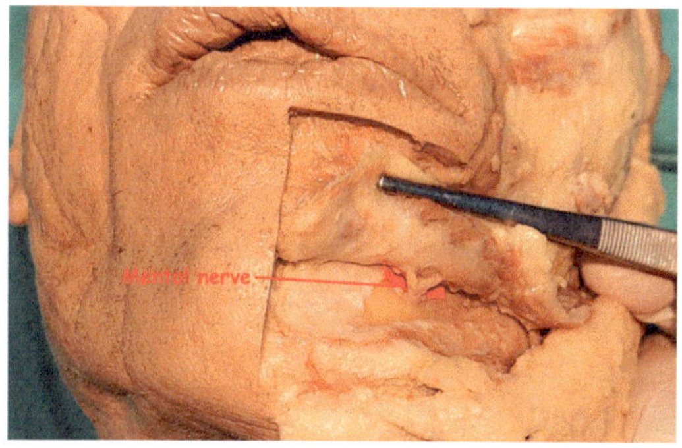


**Fig. 11** The mental nerve in cadaver

### Complications [8, 10, 16, 20]

- Bleeding (if adequate compression is not provided)
- Swelling, redness, and bruising on the skin
- Alopecia and skin atrophy (steroid use and its subcutaneous spread)
- Compression neuropathy (inserting the needle into the foramen and injecting)
- Neuritis (especially for neurolytic injections)
- Infection (rare)
- Allergic reaction to the injectate
- Globe injury

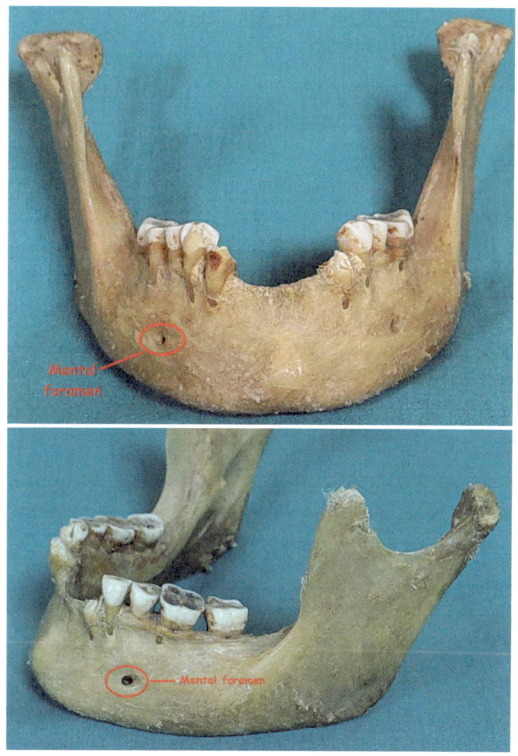


**Fig. 12** Mental foramen in the skull

## Mental Nerve Block

### Mental Nerve Anatomy

The mental nerve is one of the terminal branches of the mandibular division (CN V3) of the trigeminal nerve and provides ipsilateral sensory innervation to the chin and lower lip (Fig. 11) [1].

The mandibular nerve is both sensory and motor [1]. It exits the skull via the foramen ovale and enters the infratemporal fossa [21]. Then it gives three branches: the auriculotemporal nerve, the inferior alveolar nerve, and the lingual nerve [21]. The inferior alveolar nerve crosses the mandibular foramen and travels anteriorly in the mandibular canal [12]. Then it crosses the mental foramen, and when its terminal branch emerges, it is called the mental nerve. After ascending to the mental region, it proceeds deep into the depressor labii inferioris muscle [12].

Mental foramen lies on the mandibular bone, and it is approximately 13 mm above the inferior border of the mandible and 20–25 mm lateral to the midline (Fig. 12) [22]. It is nearly at the level of the second premolar teeth.

## Ultrasound-Guided Mental Nerve Block

### Indications

Mental nerve block is useful in the diagnosis and treatment of painful conditions in areas sensed by the mental nerve [4, 8, 9, 21]:

- Trigeminal neuralgia and neuropathy (V3 distribution)
- Acute herpes zoster and post-herpetic neuralgia (V3 distribution)
- Mental nerve neuropathy (numb chin syndrome) and nerve entrapment
  - Trauma/fractures of the mandible
  - Tumors of the oral cavity or mandible
  - Dental pathologies
  - Foraminal stenosis due to Paget's disease
- Diagnosis of trigger points and hyperalgesic zones in the mental region
- Providing surgical anesthesia or postoperative analgesia in the innervation area of the mental nerve

### Ultrasound-Guided Technique

The patient is placed in the supine position. The mental foramen is identified by palpation with the index finger at the mandible (approximately 13 mm above the inferior border of the mandible, 2.5 cm lateral to midline, or at the mid-pupillary line) [22]. The skin covering the foramen is cleaned with an antiseptic solution and prepped in a sterile fashion. On ultrasound, the bone structure is typically shown as hyperechoic (bright) linear lines, and the deep tissue behind them as hypoechoic (dark) [11]. A high-frequency linear or hockey stick transducer is placed along the mental foramen in an oblique plane (the lateral side is up and the medial side is down) (Fig. 13). The mental foramen is visualized as a bony defect or discontinuity on the hyperechoic mandible [14]. Then the mental nerve and artery (using color Doppler mode) are identified in the notch. The 25–27 gauge, 5 cm blunt-tipped nerve block needle is placed toward the mental foramen in the in-plane technique, lateral to the medial direction (Fig. 14). After touching the bone, the tip is slightly withdrawn. Following negative aspiration, 2–3 ml of local anesthetic solution

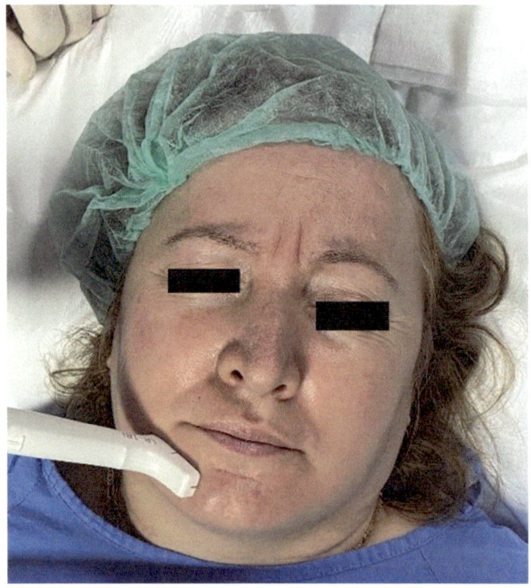

**Fig. 13** Probe placement in ultrasound-guided mental nerve block

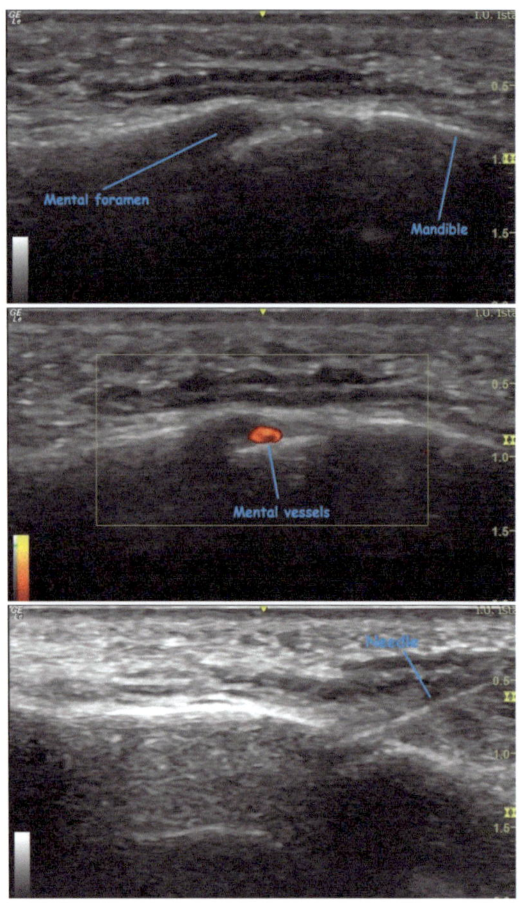


**Fig. 14** Ultrasound-guided mental nerve block

(bupivacaine 0.5% or lidocaine 2% with or without corticosteroid) is injected. In order not to cause mechanical damage to the mental nerve with the tip of the needle or compressive damage to the mental nerve with the injectate, placement of the tip of the needle in the foramen should be avoided [8, 10, 14]. After the block procedure, pressure should be applied to the injection site to prevent bleeding and hematoma formation [8].

The blockade provides anesthesia in the dermatome area of the nerve. It allows diagnostically to determine whether the supraorbital nerve is present in the pain pathway. Or therapeutically, it provides analgesia in the relevant area. Mostly the resulting analgesia is short-lived and ends when the effect of the local anesthetic solution on the nerve disappears. However, longer-lasting effects can be obtained by methods such as adding steroids to the solution, making repetitive blocks, and using thermal radiofrequency ablation, cryoablation, or chemical neurolysis [21].

## Complications [8, 10, 21]

- Bleeding (if adequate compression is not provided)
- Swelling, redness, and bruising on the skin
- Alopecia and skin atrophy (steroid use and its subcutaneous spread)
- Compression neuropathy (inserting the needle into the foramen and injecting)
- Neuritis (especially for neurolytic injections)
- Infection (rare)
- Allergic reaction to the injectate

## References


1. Dalley AF, Agur AMR. Moore's clinically oriented anatomy. 9th ed. Philadelphia: Walters Kluwer; 2023.
2. Lin C-S, Cheng J. Trigeminal nerve blocks and neurolysis. In: Manchikanti L, Kaye AD, Falco FJE, Hirsch JA, editors. Essentials of interventional techniques in managing chronic pain. Springer; 2018. p. 451–61.
3. Spinner D, Kirschner JS. Accuracy of ultrasound-guided superficial trigeminal nerve blocks using methylene blue in cadavers. Pain Med. 2012;13(11):1469–73. https://doi.org/10.1111/j.1526-4637.2012.01480.x.
4. Costandi S, Costandi J, Souzdalnitski D, Narouze SN. Peripheral nerve block for the management of headache and face pain. In: Narouze SN, editor. Interventional management of head and face pain nerve blocks and beyond. New York: Springer; 2014. p. 17–27.
5. Justiz R. Supraorbital nerve entrapment: face. In: Trescot AM, editor. Peripheral nerve entrapments, clinical diagnosis and management. Switzerland: Springer; 2016. p. 185–96.
6. Tsutsumi S, Ono H, Ishii H, Yasumoto Y. Visualization of the supraorbital notch/foramen using magnetic resonance imaging. J Clin Neurosci. 2019;62:212–5. https://doi.org/10.1016/j.jocn.2019.01.005.
7. Fallucco M, Janis JE, Hagan RR. The anatomical morphology of the supraorbital notch: clinical relevance to the surgical treatment of migraine headaches. Plast Reconstr Surg. 2012;130:1227–33.
8. Waldman SD. Atlas of interventional pain management. 4th ed. Philadelphia: Elsevier, Saunders; 2015.
9. Jankovic D, Tsui BCH. Trigeminal nerve. In: Jankovic D, Peng P, editors. Regional nerve blocks in anesthesia and pain therapy, traditional and ultrasound-guided techniques. 4th ed. Cham: Springer; 2015. p. 133–60.
10. Kissoon NR. Blockade of the nerves of the head and face. In: Deer TR, Pope JE, Lamer TJ, Provenzano D, editors. Deer's treatment of pain, an illustrated guide for practitioners. Springer; 2019. p. 297–312.
11. Tsui BC. Ultrasound imaging to localize foramina for superficial trigeminal nerve block. Can J Anaesth. 2009;56(9):704–6.
12. Allam AE, Khalil AAF, Eltawab BA, Wu WT, Chang KV. Ultrasound-guided intervention for treatment of trigeminal neuralgia: an updated review of anatomy and techniques. Pain Res Manag. 2018;2018:5480728. https://doi.org/10.1155/2018/5480728.
13. Garg RK, Lee KS, Kohn SC, Baskaya MK, Afifi AM. Can sonography distinguish a supraorbital notch from a foramen? J Ultrasound Med. 2015;34(11):2089–91. https://doi.org/10.7863/ultra.14.12015.
14. Waldman SD. Comprehensive atlas of ultrasound-guided pain management injection techniques. 1st ed. Philadelphia: Lippincott Williams & Wilkins; 2014.
15. Barnard NA, Bainton R. Bradycardia and the trigeminal nerve. J Craniomaxillofac Surg. 1990;18(8):359–60. https://doi.org/10.1016/s1010-5182(05)80056-3.
16. Justiz R, Kaplan ED. Infraorbital nerve entrapment. In: Trescot AM, editor. Peripheral nerve entrapments, clinical diagnosis and management. Switzerland: Springer; 2016. p. 197–204.
17. Aggarwal A, Kaur H, Gupta T, Tubbs RS, Sahni D, Batra YK, Sondekoppam RV. Anatomical study of the infraorbital foramen: a basis for successful infraorbital nerve block. Clin Anat. 2015;28(6):753–60. https://doi.org/10.1002/ca.22558.

18. Shin KJ, Lee SH, Park MG, Shin HJ, Lee AG. Location of the accessory infraorbital foramen with reference to external landmarks and its clinical implications. Sci Rep. 2020;10(1):8566. https://doi.org/10.1038/s41598-020-65330-4.
19. Lim SM, Park HL, Moon HY, Kang KH, Kang H, Baek CH, Jung YH, Kim JY, Koo GH, Shin HY. Ultrasound-guided infraorbital nerve pulsed radiofrequency treatment for intractable postherpetic neuralgia – a case report. Korean J Pain. 2013;26(1):84–8. https://doi.org/10.3344/kjp.2013.26.1.84.
20. Saeedi OJ, Wang H, Blomquist PH. Penetrating globe injury during infraorbital nerve block. Arch Otolaryngol Head Neck Surg. 2011;137:396–7.
21. Rose SE, Gulati A. Mental nerve entrapment. In: Trescot AM, editor. Peripheral nerve entrapments, clinical diagnosis and management. Switzerland: Springer; 2016. p. 229–40.
22. Ebrahim Laher A, Mahomed Z. The ultrasonographic determination of the position of the mental foramen and its relation to hard tissue landmarks. Acta Med Acad. 2016;45(1):51–60.

# GON, LON, TON Blocks

Manfred Greher

## Introduction

The three occipital nerves in the human body that innervate the posterior skin areas of the head partially including the ears are the greater occipital nerve (GON), the lesser occipital nerve (LON), and the third occipital nerve (TON). Local anesthetic blocks of these nerves play an important role in the successful management of different primary and secondary headache disorders as well as neck pain and should therefore be well-known to pain specialists and be part of their invasive treatment spectrum. Selective ultrasound-guided block techniques that offer many advantages compared to blind infiltrations were first published in 2006 for the TON [1] and in 2010 for the GON [2] by our study group. Sonographic visualization of the LON was subsequently described in 2015 by another Austrian group [3].

## Anatomy and Innervation Areas

The three occipital nerves all arise from the C2 and C3 spinal nerves, innervating the posterior scalp together as a group with a lot of interconnecting fibers. Thorough knowledge of their anatomical origin and course is key to understanding the pathophysiology of nerve compression syndromes as well as the essentials of visualizing the nerves with ultrasound. Interestingly, the density of the peripheral afferent nerve fibers is typically higher in the lateral occipital regions compared to the median area, leaving a nerve-rarified zone in the shape of an inverted triangle on top of the external occipital protuberance [4]. Figure 1 shows a typical distribution of the occipital sensory innervation areas.

M. Greher (✉)
Department of Anesthesiology,
Herz-Jesu Krankenhaus GmbH, Wien, Austria
e-mail: manfred.greher@kh-herzjesu.at

## Greater Occipital Nerve

The GON is a big sensory branch that arises from the medial branch of the primary dorsal ramus of the C2 spinal nerve and can infrequently get contributing fibers from the C3 dorsal ramus. After emerging below the posterior arch of the atlas and above the lamina of the axis, it curls around the inferior border of the obliquus capitis inferior muscle (OCIM) in a cephalad direction from lateral to medial to reach a position on top of this muscle sandwiched between the OCIM and the semispinalis capitis muscle (SSCM) in the roof of the suboccipital triangle. Only in very rare cases is the GON found within the OCIM. The OCIM connects the spinous process of C2 with the transverse process of C1,



T. Akkaya, A. Cömert (eds.), *Practical Guide for Pain Interventions: Head and Neck Sonoanatomy*,
https://doi.org/10.1007/978-3-031-88773-4_7

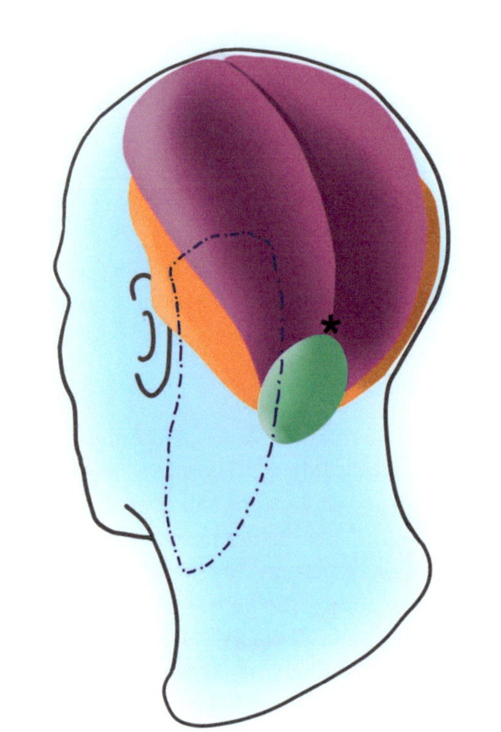

**Fig. 1** Typical cutaneous sensory innervation areas of the occipital nerves (GON magenta, LON orange, TON green) and projected pain areas in C2/3 facet joint derived pain (area marked by semicolon line), asterisk = greater occipital protuberance

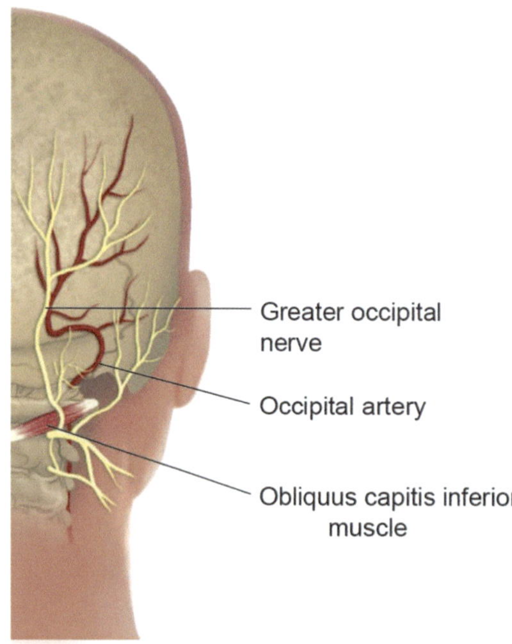


**Fig. 2** GON curling around the OCIM joining the artery at the superior nuchal line

running from medio-caudal to latero-cranial, and is the important sonographic landmark for the proximal GON block technique at the level of C2. From there, the GON pierces the medial head of the SSCM in the majority of cases, then the aponeurotic fibrous layer of the trapezius muscle (TM) and sometimes the splenius capitis muscle (SCM) and reaches the subcutis at the superior nuchal line medial to the occipital artery (OA). This is the location for the distal GON block. While branching, it further ascends cranially with the OA. The GON innervates the posterior hemicranial part of the scalp up to the vertex and variable parts of the retroauricular skin. Due to this complicated course of the GON in relation to several muscular planes, there are potential sources of nerve compression on its way to the scalp (Fig. 2).

## Lesser Occipital Nerve

The LON is the most cranial nerve of the cervical plexus and arises from the ventral rami of the C2 and C3 spinal nerves. The LON winds around the posterior margin of the sternocleidomastoid muscle (SCMM) and runs cranially to the parietooccipital region along this landmark line. The LON penetrates the deep cervical fascia on top of the levator scapulae muscle (LSM) close to the cranium. The course is quite variable, and branching can occur early so that identification with ultrasound is best accomplished starting at the posterior border of the SCMM caudal to the mastoid. The LON sends communicating branches to the GON and innervates the skin lateral to the area of the GON behind the ear. Most commonly, the LON provides sensory supply to the superior ear and the mastoid area, whereas the great auricular nerve (GAN), which also originates from the cervical plexus, innervates the inferior part of the ear and a part of the preauricular area. Sometimes, however, in the case of a small GAN, the LON can provide the dominant sensory supply of the ear [5].

## Third Occipital Nerve

The TON is different from the GON and LON because—additionally to innervating a small skin area medially below the superior nuchal line—it also provides sensory innervation to the C2/3 zygapophyseal (=facet) joint and motor innervation to parts of the SSCM. The TON is the superficial medial branch of the dorsal ramus of the C3 spinal nerve. The deep medial branch of the C3 spinal nerve is smaller than the TON and runs caudally to innervate the C3/4 facet joint together with the C4 medial branch. While each facet joint receives fibers from the medial branches above and below, the C2/3 facet joint is the only one that exclusively gets sensory supply from a single nerve, which is the TON. C2/3 facet joint-derived pain is typically referred in the neck/head region as shown in Fig. 1. The TON travels on top of the dorsolateral surface of the C2/3 joint, as opposed to the other medial branches that are located between two joints in the "valleys." The C2/3 joint therefore is the key sonographic landmark to locate and block the TON proximally, as needed for a C2/3 facet joint block. It can also frequently be identified just medial to the GON on top of the OCIM at the level of C2.

The TON sends communicating fibers to the contralateral TON in two-thirds of cases inferior to the external occipital protuberance [6]. Further peripherally and cranially, the TON perforates the SCM, the TM, and the SSCM and communicates with the GON.

Under perfect conditions, an ultrasound image parallel to the OCIM at the C2 level can show all three nerves in a single sonographic plane (Figs. 3 and 4).

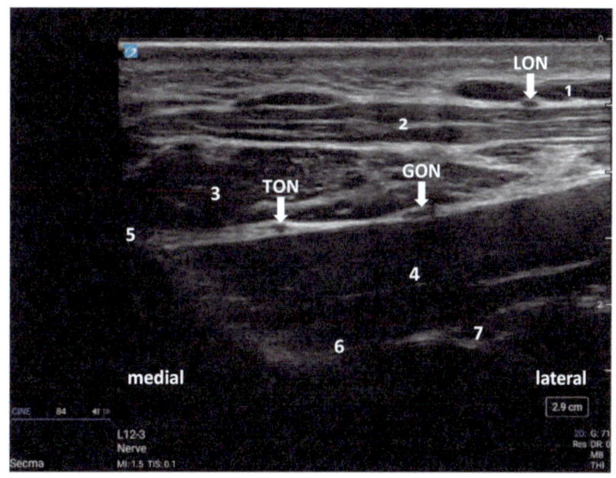


**Fig. 3** Transverse ultrasound image showing all 3 occipital nerves in a single plane, 1 = SCMM, 2 = SCM, 3 = SSCM, 4 = OCIM, 5 = C2 spinous process, 6 = C2 lamina, 7 = C2 dorsal root ganglion

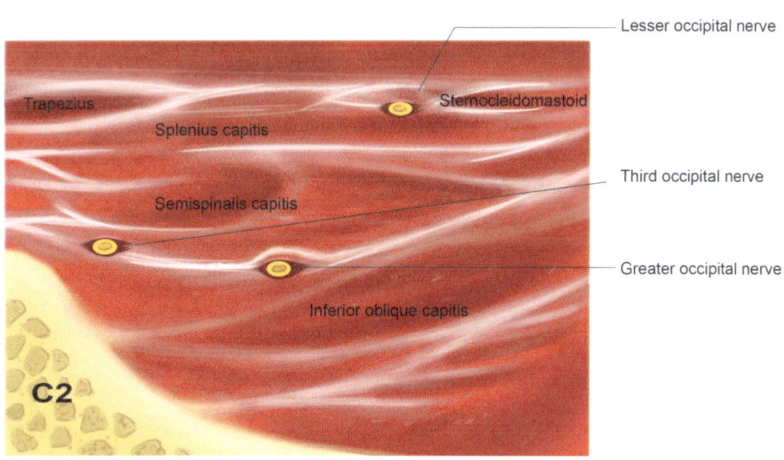


**Fig. 4** Anatomical drawing corresponding to Fig. 3

## Indications and Evidence for Blocks

According to the recent third edition of the International Classification of Headache Disorders (ICHD-3), there are more than 200 types of headaches in 14 main groups [7].

Occipital neuralgia is described as unilateral or bilateral paroxysmal, shooting, or stabbing pain in the posterior part of the scalp, in the distribution(s) of the greater, lesser, and/or third occipital nerves, sometimes accompanied by diminished sensation or dysesthesia in the affected area and commonly associated with tenderness over the involved nerve(s). Diagnostic criteria include positive local anesthetic (LA) blocks of the affected nerve(s).

Blocks of the occipital nerves have been proven effective in randomized controlled trials and cohort studies for several primary and secondary headaches like cluster headaches, acute and chronic migraine, occipital neuralgia, and chronic daily headache [8]. Additional indications like cervicogenic-, posttraumatic/surgical- or post-dural puncture headache have been included in another expert consensus recommendation with lower levels of evidence [9].

Pain reduction after endovascular therapy of cranial aneurysms has recently been reported in two cases after bilateral GON blocks [10].

Finally, C2/3 facet joint-derived pain, which is especially common after a whiplash injury, can be diagnosed and treated either with intraarticular infiltrations or specific TON blocks [1]. If two LA test blocks provide significant but only temporary relief, radiofrequency denervation is commonly recommended and can also be facilitated with ultrasound guidance [11].

## Possible Mechanisms of Action

The exact underlying mechanisms of why GON blocks are clinically effective in different types of primary headaches are still poorly understood. However, the so-called trigeminocervical complex in the spinal cord at the level of C1/2 seems to play an important role. Converging trigeminal and occipital fibers perform a crucial functional neuroanatomical connection with substantial intertalk in that region, that could explain observed clinical effects by blocking afferent occipital nerve fibers. Inhibition of trigeminal nociceptive activity is likely to occur after a GON block [12]. Recently, calcitonin-gene-related-peptide (CGRP)-targeted antibodies have been approved for migraine prophylaxis since CGRP was identified as a key player in chronic migraine. Interestingly, GON blocks were also found to significantly suppress CGRP levels in a clinical investigation, implying a potential role for CGRP in the mechanism of GON block action [13].

## Advantages of Ultrasound Guidance

In comparison to superficial landmark-based "blind" LA blocks of the three occipital nerves, ultrasound guidance adds specificity, efficacy, and safety by direct visualization of the target nerves, adjacent tissues, the needle tip, and LA spread. Occasionally, blind infiltrations can lead to disastrous complications [14]. A study comparing blind GON blocks at the superior nuchal line with ultrasound-guided blocks at the C2 level found higher clinical efficacy for the latter [15]. Moreover, anatomical variabilities of the tiny occipital nerves can best be detected with today's high-frequency ultrasound transducers. Compared to ultrasound, fluoroscopy cannot visualize nerves but only bony landmarks and cannot prevent but only detect inadvertent vascular punctures. Ionizing radiation is totally avoided under ultrasound, which is an advantage for both patient and physician and makes it the first choice during pregnancy. A randomized comparison found similar success rates but improved efficiency for ultrasound compared to fluoroscopy in TON blocks [16]. Modern ultrasound devices have recently become miniaturized, highly portable, and attached to smartphones or tablet PCs; the applicability increases enormously.

## Block Technique and Sonoanatomy

For blocks of all three nerves, high-frequency linear transducers are used. For a GON block at a greater distance from the skin, decreasing the imaging frequency while increasing the far gain can be helpful.

## Greater Occipital Nerve

The patient is placed in a lateral decubitus position with the side to be blocked upwards. The physician is standing behind the patient's neck, and the patient and the physician are facing the ultrasound machine on the other side of the bed. The patient's neck is in anteflexion, the head supported by a small pillow below the ear to keep the cervical spine line straight. The mastoid process is palpated with the index finger, and the lateral end of the ultrasound transducer is placed just dorsal to it. The medial end of the ultrasound transducer is placed 2 cm more caudal than the lateral end and close to the midline. This almost transverse but slightly oblique transducer position is now in the majority of cases exactly parallel to and on top of the OCIM, which is more hypoechogenic compared to the muscles overlying it.

On the medial side of the image, the C2 spinous process with bone shadows behind can be recognized; on the lateral side and deep to the lamina of C2, blood flow within the vertebral artery can be identified with color Doppler. On top of the OCIM and sandwiched between this muscle and the SSCM, the hypoechogenic GON can be found. Deep to the C2 lamina, the C2 dorsal root ganglion can often be visualized. Lowering the pressure on the transducer together with color- or power Doppler mode helps to rule out compressed veins in the vicinity of the GON. Often, the significantly smaller TON can be identified slightly medial to the GON on the OCIM or in the SSCM. Adjacent to the dorsal border of the SCMM, the LON can sometimes be identified in the same image (Fig. 4).

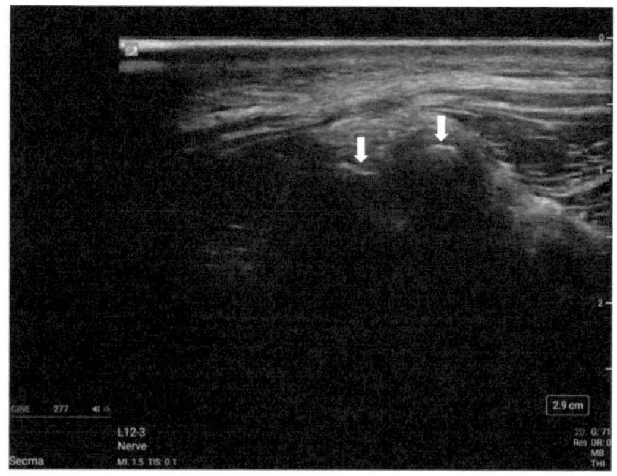


**Fig. 5** Transverse ultrasound image showing the bifid spinous process of C2 (arrows)

If the "quick" technique of palpating the mastoid process as described above does not result in the right ultrasound plane with the necessary sonoanatomic landmarks, another procedure can be recommended: starting with the transducer transversely in the midline on top of the occiput and sliding down caudally shows the arch of the atlas first and the bifid spinous process of the C2 vertebra second (Fig. 5). This is exactly where the OCIM attaches medially. Moving the transducer laterally and rotating the lateral end of the transducer approximately 2 cm cranially places it exactly parallel to the OCIM and shows the GON on top of this muscle.

The block can be performed either with an out-of-plane (needle caudal to the transducer, Fig. 6) or an in-plane (needle lateral to the transducer, Fig. 7) needle insertion technique. A sharp beveled 4 cm 25G needle attached to an extension line with a 5 ml syringe is suitable in most cases. With the needle tip lateral to the GON and after a negative aspiration test, 1.5–3 ml of LA are injected slowly around the GON (Fig. 8).

Figure 9 shows the transducer position for this proximal block technique at C2 in comparison to the "classical" distal block site at the superior nuchal line, where GON visualization is far more difficult due to the short distance between the transducer and target [2].

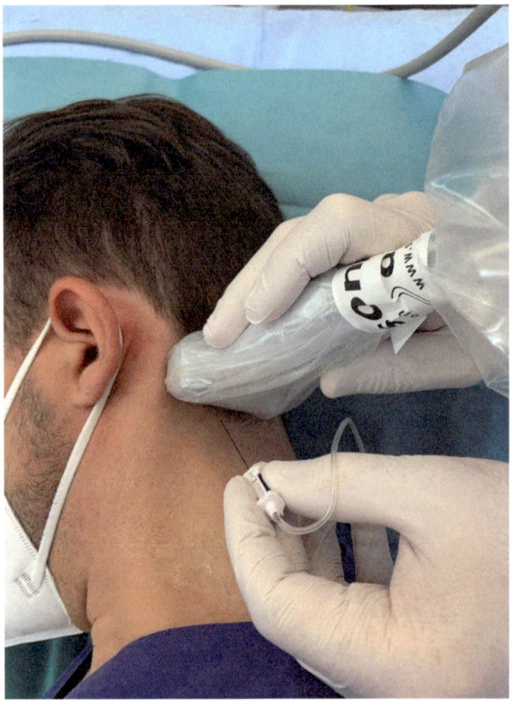

Fig. 6 GON block procedure OOP

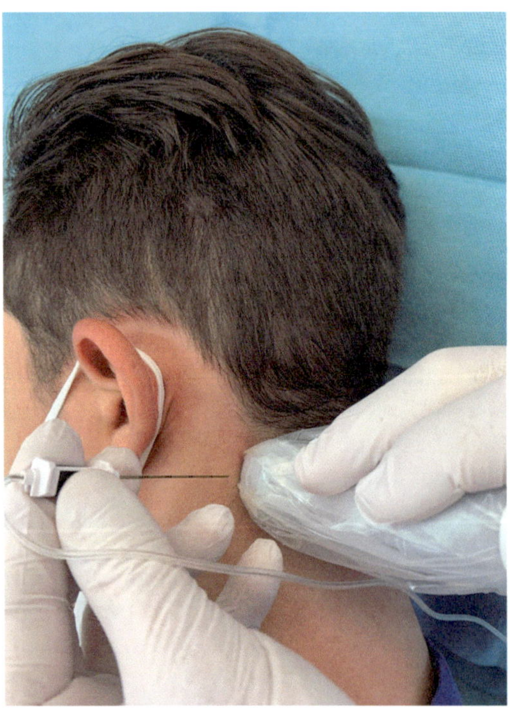

Fig. 7 GON block procedure IP

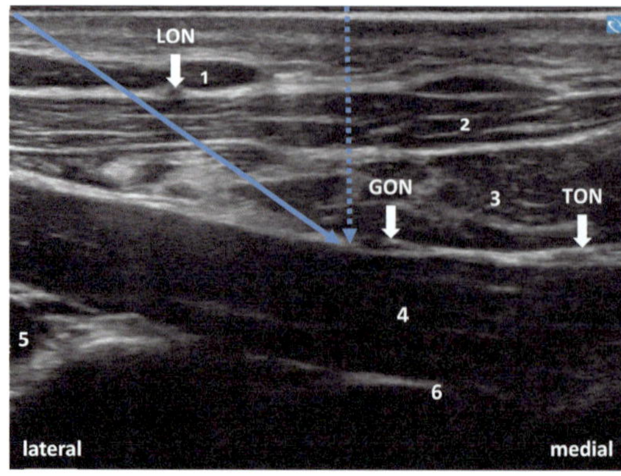


**Fig. 8** Transverse ultrasound GON block image showing OOP (dotted blue arrow) and IP (continuous blue arrow) needle directions, 1 = SCMM, 2 = SCM, 3 = SSCM, 4 = OCIM, 5 = vertebral artery, 6 = C2 lamina

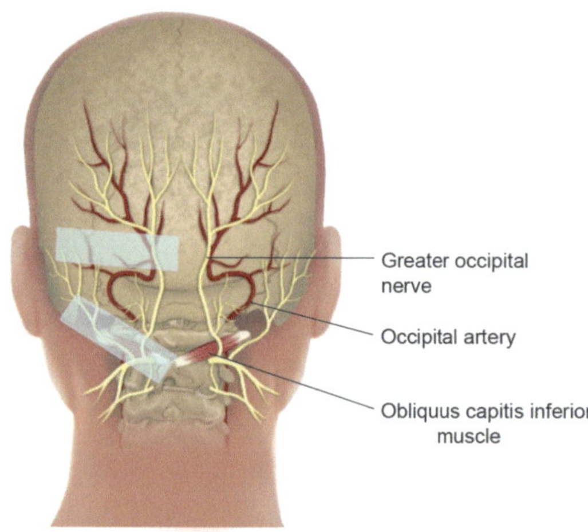


**Fig. 9** Anatomical drawing showing the ultrasound transducer positions for the proximal GON block at C2 (lower green box) and the distal at the superior nuchal line (upper green box)

## Lesser Occipital Nerve

The patient is placed in a lateral decubitus position with the side to be blocked upwards. The physician is standing behind the patient's neck, and the patient and the physician are facing the ultrasound machine on the other side of the bed. The patient's neck can be flexed; the head can be supported by a small pillow below the ear. After palpation of the SCMM's dorsal border, the

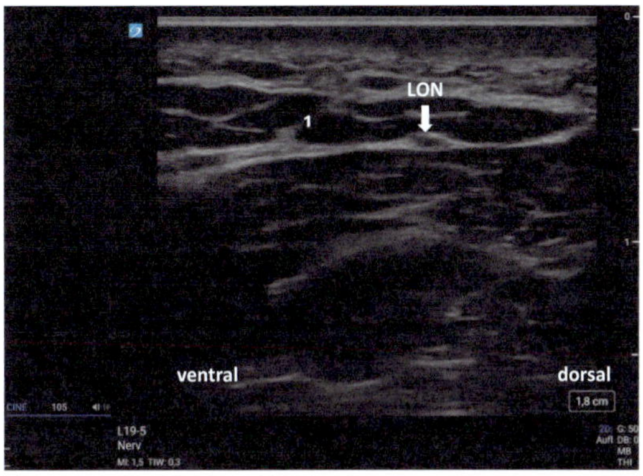


**Fig. 10** Transverse ultrasound image showing the LON, 1 = SCMM

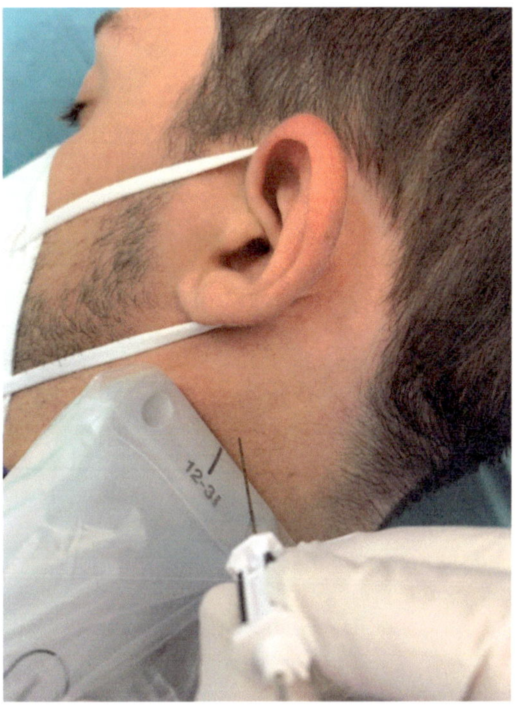

**Fig. 11** LON block procedure OOP

transducer is placed perpendicular to the muscle in a transverse orientation approximately 3–5 cm caudal to the mastoid process. By sliding the transducer from the caudal to the cranial and back, a small hypoechogenic nerve deep and dorsal to the SCMM is identified (Fig. 10).

The block can be performed either with an out-of-plane (needle cranial to the transducer, Fig. 11) or an in-plane (needle dorsal to the

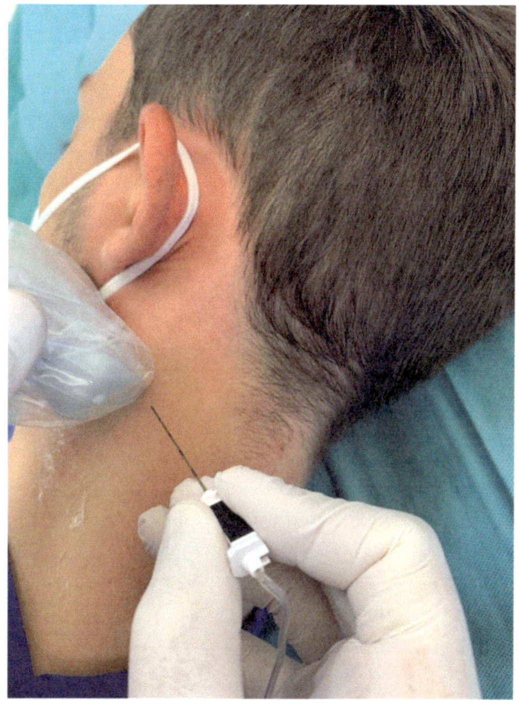

**Fig. 12** LON block procedure IP

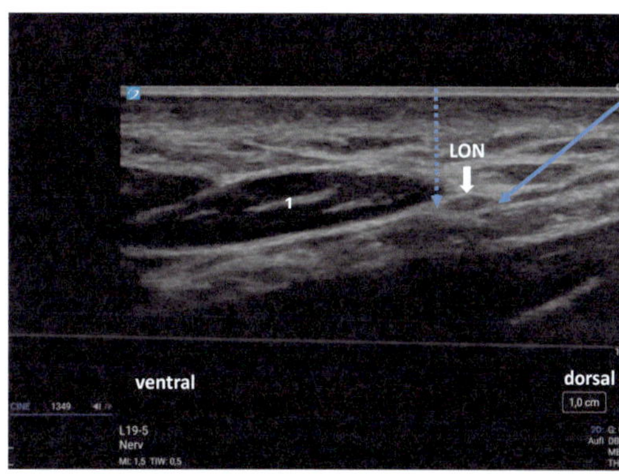


**Fig. 13** Transverse ultrasound LON block image showing OOP (dotted blue arrow) and IP (continuous blue arrow) needle directions, 1 = SCMM

transducer, Fig. 12) needle insertion technique. A sharp beveled 4 cm 25G needle attached to an extension line with a 5 ml syringe is suitable in most cases. With the needle tip close to the LON and after a negative aspiration test, 1–3 ml of LA is injected slowly around the LON (Fig. 13).

## Third Occipital Nerve

The patient is placed in a lateral decubitus position with the side to be blocked upwards. The physician is standing in front of the patient, facing the ultrasound machine on the other side of the bed. The patient's neck is in a neutral position, the head supported by a small pillow below the ear to keep the cervical spine line straight. The mastoid process is palpated with the index finger, and the cranial end of the ultrasound transducer is placed immediately caudal to it with a longitudinal orientation. The ultrasound image now shows a bony wave line of the facet joints with the articular pillows on top. The C2/3 joint is identified as the first one visible most cranially. On top of the C2/3 joint, the TON can be located and blocked. The block should be performed out of a plane (needle anterior to the transducer, Fig. 14) from ventral to dorsal. Thus, block safety is increased by avoiding potentially vulnerable structures like the vertebral artery or the nerve roots ventral to the articulations. A sharp beveled 4 cm 25G needle attached to an extension line with a 2 ml syringe is used. With the needle tip close to the TON and after a negative aspiration test, 0.3–0.5 ml of LA for diagnostic blocks are injected slowly around the nerve (Fig. 15). If localization of the joint line gets difficult in the longitudinal view, rotating the transducer in the transverse view and back can be helpful.

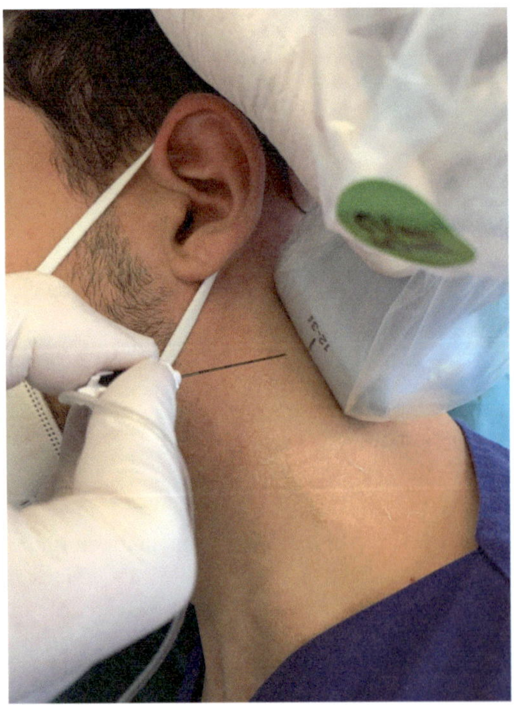

**Fig. 14** TON block procedure OOP

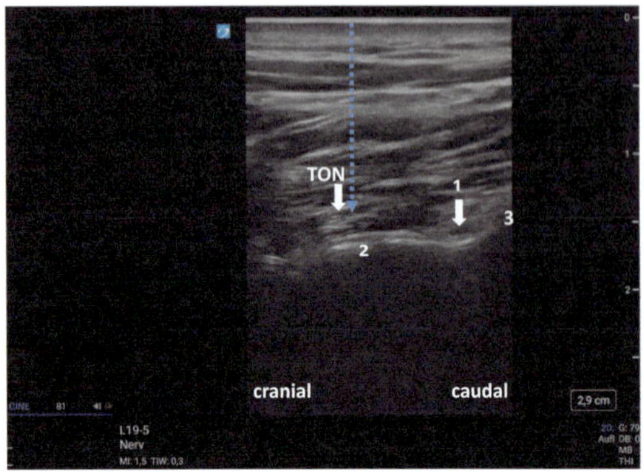


**Fig. 15** Longitudinal ultrasound TON block image showing OOP (dotted blue arrow) needle direction, 1 = C3 medial branch, 2 = C2/3 facet joint, 3 = C3/4 facet joint

## Clinical Tips and Tricks

Bilateral blocks are feasible and can best be performed with the patient in a prone or sitting position. One should be aware that transient dizziness and vertigo are more common after bilateral occipital nerve blocks.

Ultrasound-guided occipital nerve blocks are very safe and effective [17]. However, careful prevention of inadvertent vascular injection is important. Low transducer pressure to visualize collapsed veins, color- or power Doppler examinations, and aspiration on the syringe before injection should be performed on a regular basis. Reliable sonographic visualization of LA spread around the nerve in real time should always be the aim.

Most used types of LA are lidocaine 1–2%, bupivacaine 0.25–0.5%, and ropivacaine 0.2–0.5%.

Mixing steroids like dexamethasone 4 mg with LA is a common practice to prolong the block duration and provide additional analgesic properties.

If refractory pain recurs even after a series of blocks, cryoanalgesia, radiofrequency, neurolysis, or botulinum toxin injections are further options and can also be facilitated by ultrasound guidance.

Cutaneous branches of the suboccipital nerve and the spinal accessory nerve are present additionally in certain cases and can send communicating fibers to the other occipital nerves.

## Literature


1. Eichenberger U, Greher M, Kapral S, Marhofer P, Wiest R, Remonda L, Bogduk N, Curatolo M. Sonographic visualization and ultrasound-guided block of the third occipital nerve: prospective for a new method to diagnose C2–C3 zygapophysial joint pain. Anesthesiology. 2006;104(2):303–8.
2. Greher M, Moriggl B, Curatolo M, Kirchmair L, Eichenberger U. Sonographic visualization and ultrasound-guided blockade of the greater occipital nerve: a comparison of two selective techniques confirmed by anatomical dissection. Br J Anaesth. 2010;104(5):637–42.
3. Platzgummer H, Moritz T, Gruber GM, Pivec C, Wöber C, Bodner G, Lieba-Samal D. The lesser occipital nerve visualized by high-resolution sonography--normal and initial suspect findings. Cephalalgia. 2015;35(9):816–24.
4. Kwon HJ, Kim HS, Jehoon O, Kang HJ, Won JY, Yang HM, Kim SH, Choi YJ. Anatomical analysis of the distribution patterns of occipital cutaneous nerves and the clinical implications for pain management. J Pain Res. 2018;25(11):2023–31.
5. Pantaloni M, Sullivan P. Relevance of the lesser occipital nerve in facial rejuvenation surgery. Plast Reconstr Surg. 2000;105(7):2594–9.
6. Tubbs RS, Mortazavi MM, Loukas M, D'Antoni AV, Shoja MM, Chern JJ, Cohen-Gadol AA. Anatomical study of the third occipital nerve and its potential role in occipital headache/neck pain following midline dissections of the craniocervical junction. J Neurosurg Spine. 2011;15(1):71–5.
7. Headache Classification Committee of the International Headache Society (IHS). The international classification of headache disorders, 3rd edition (beta version). Cephalalgia. 2013;33(9):629–808.
8. Fernandes L, Randall M, Idrovo L. Peripheral nerve blocks for headache disorders. Pract Neurol. 2021;21:30–5.
9. Blumenfeld A, Ashkenazi A, Napchan U, Bender SD, Klein BC, Berliner R, Ailani J, Schim J, Friedman DI, Charleston L 4th, Young WB, Robertson CE, Dodick DW, Silberstein SD, Robbins MS. Expert consensus recommendations for the performance of peripheral nerve blocks for headaches-a narrative review. Headache. 2013;53(3):437–46.
10. Doğan R, Pınar HU, Karaca Ö, Karakoç F. Ultrasound-guided bilateral greater occipital nerve block on headache seen after endovascular treatment of ruptured or unruptured intracranial aneurysms: a case report. Agri. 2020;32(4):223–7.
11. Siegenthaler A, Eichenberger U, Curatolo M. A shortened radiofrequency denervation method for cervical zygapophysial joint pain based on ultrasound localization of the nerves. Pain Med. 2011;12(12):1703–9.
12. Hoffmann J, Mehnert J, Koo EM, May A. Greater occipital nerve block modulates nociceptive signals within the trigeminocervical complex. J Neurol Neurosurg Psychiatry. 2021;92(12):1335–40.
13. Abbas A, Moustafa R, Shalash A, Haroun M, Amin R, Borham S, Elsadek A, Helmy S. Serum CGRP changes following ultrasound-guided bilateral greater-occipital-nerve block. Neurol Int. 2022;14(1):199–206.
14. Sprenger T, Seifert CL. Coma after greater occipital nerve blockade in a patient with previous posterior fossa surgery. Headache. 2013;53(3):548–50.
15. Kissoon NR, O'Brien TG, Bendel MA, Eldrige JS, Hagedorn JM, Mauck WD, Moeschler SM, Olatoye OO, Pittelkow TP, Watson JC, Pingree MJ. Comparative effectiveness of landmark-guided greater occipital nerve (GON) block at the superior nuchal line versus ultrasound-guided GON block at the level of C2: a randomized clinical trial (RCT). Clin J Pain. 2022;38(4):271–8.
16. Finlayson RJ, Etheridge JP, Vieira L, Gupta G, Tran DQ. A randomized comparison between ultrasound- and fluoroscopy-guided third occipital nerve block. Reg Anesth Pain Med. 2013;38(3):212–7.
17. Chowdhury D, Datta D, Mundra A. Role of greater occipital nerve block in headache disorders: a narrative review. Neurol India. 2021;69(Supplement): S228–56.

# Great Auricular Nerve Block

Marko Konschake

## Background

Peripheral nerve blocks or decompression surgery for head and neck nerve trigger sites has demonstrated effectiveness in addressing, e.g., migraine headaches resulting from peripheral nerve compression. Unlike traditional migraines, peripheral nerve compression headaches are believed to have an extracranial origin, involving compression of nerves outside the skull. These compression sites can involve bony or fascial structures (e.g., supraorbital foramen or notch/supraorbital nerve), blood vessels (e.g., superficial temporal artery/auriculotemporal nerve; occipital artery/greater occipital nerve), and muscles (e.g., corrugator muscle/supratrochlear nerve). Extensive evidence supports the use of blocks, surgery, and targeted botulinum toxin injections in relieving headaches at these known trigger sites [1, 3, 5].

However, despite decompression procedures targeting known trigger sites, there is a subset of patients who continue to experience inadequately treated symptoms, particularly postauricular and posterior temporal pain. These patients specifically describe focal pain centered around the back of the ear, following the course of the postauricular sulcus. Based on our observations, the literature proposes that these patients may be experiencing headache symptoms due to compression of the great auricular nerve (GAN), also known as the nervus auricularis magnus [2, 5, 7].

While the anatomical pathway of the GAN has been established, emerging from the ventral cervical rami C2 and C3 at Erb's point (known as the "nerve point of neck"), traveling cranially along the sternocleidomastoid muscle (SCM), and dividing into anterior and posterior branches beneath the posterior aspect of the earlobe, an anatomical study has investigated the GAN's course in relation to potential compression sites contributing to peripheral nerve compression headaches [5].

The use of GAN blocks has gained prominence in the fields of otolaryngology, plastic surgery, and pain management. These blocks have been applied for diagnostic purposes, therapeutic interventions, and as an adjunct to regional anesthesia techniques. The diagnostic value of GAN blocks lies in their ability to confirm or rule out the involvement of the GAN in patients with localized pain or sensory disturbances in the innervated regions. By selectively anesthetizing the GAN, clinicians can assess whether the patient experiences pain relief or sensory improvement. This diagnostic information aids in the differential diagnosis and subsequent management decisions. Additionally, GAN blocks

M. Konschake (✉)
Department of Anatomy, Histology and Embryology, Institute of Clinical and Functional Anatomy, Medical University of Innsbruck (MUI), Innsbruck, Austria
e-mail: marko.konschake@i-med.ac.at



T. Akkaya, A. Cömert (eds.), *Practical Guide for Pain Interventions: Head and Neck Sonoanatomy*,
https://doi.org/10.1007/978-3-031-88773-4_8

can be employed therapeutically to provide short-term or long-term pain relief for conditions such as postoperative pain, trigeminal neuralgia, or neuropathic pain involving the GAN distribution [4, 6, 7].

The techniques for performing GAN blocks have evolved. Initially, landmark-based techniques using palpation and anatomical landmarks were employed. However, the use of ultrasound guidance has gained popularity due to its ability to enhance accuracy and safety. Ultrasound allows real-time visualization of the GAN, adjacent structures, and the spread of local anesthetic, thereby minimizing complications and improving the success rate of the blocks [4, 6, 7].

Anatomical considerations are paramount for successful nerve blocks, and, therefore, a profound understanding of the course and variations of the GAN is crucial.

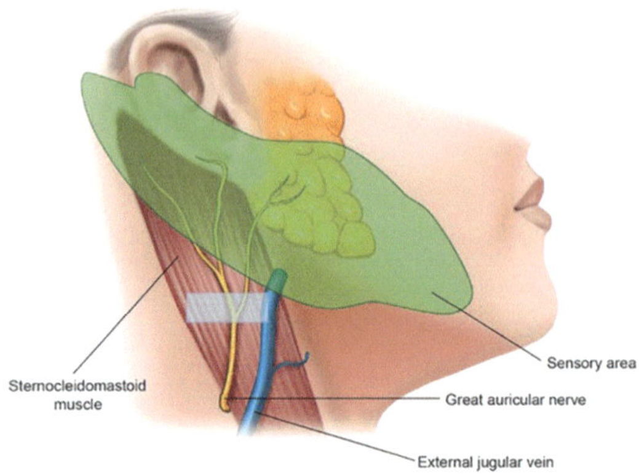


**Fig. 1** The figure gives an overview of the topographical course of the GAN and its sensory innervation area

## Topography of the Great Auricular Nerve (GAN) (Figs. 1 and 2)

The great auricular nerve (GAN) is a sensory branch of the cervical plexus, originating from the cervical spinal nerves C2 and C3. Regularly, the GAN is described as emerging from the posterior border of the sternocleidomastoid muscle (SCM) at Erb's point (also referred to as the "nerve point of neck" or better "Area nervosa") and coursing superiorly along the SCM before dividing into anterior and posterior branches. The course of the GAN begins at Erb's point with its penetration of the superficial cervical fascia, further cranially along the SCM within the superficial cervical fascia, and its branching in the anterior and posterior branches before entering the parotid gland. Anatomical studies have also revealed variations in the GAN's origin, branching patterns, and relationship with neighboring structures. These variations necessitate a meticulous approach during nerve block procedures to ensure accurate localization and optimal anesthetic delivery [5]. Possible trigger sites of the GAN during this course were: when penetrating the superficial layer of the cervical fascia (Erb's point); when entering the dense connective tissue near the anterior border of SCM (before entering the parotid gland); and when within its intraparotid course.

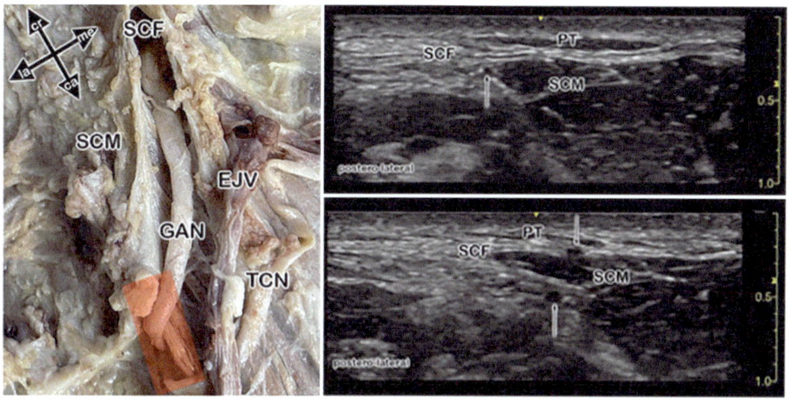


**Fig. 2** The dissection and ultrasonography of the potential site of GAN compression are depicted: Illustrating the initial location where the GAN may be compressed as it pierces the superficial cervical fascia at Erb's point. This observation was made through the utilization of ultrasound imaging and dissection performed on a body donor. The orange square represents the Erb point; black arrow indicates GAN while penetrating the SCF. SCF superficial cervical fascia, SCM sternocleidomastoid muscle, PT platysma, TCN transversuscolli nerve, EJV external jugular vein

## Ultrasonographic Approach (Fig. 2)

The ultrasonographic approach demonstrated that all possible sites of compression of the GAN could be visualized using ultrasound. The distinctive anatomical reference points for observing the GAN were as follows: Erb's Point, detectable when the platysma contracts, where the GAN intersects the back edge of the SCM. The GAN (and its branches) could be observed at the outer, upper edge of the SCM as it traverses the superficial cervical fascia and continues along its upward path on the SCM's surface until it reaches the parotid gland. The positioning of the GAN branches within the glandular structure can also be observed.

## References

1. Berchtold V, Stofferin H, Moriggl B, Brenner E, Pauzenberger R, Konschake M. Thesupraorbital region revisited: an anatomic exploration of the neurovascular bundle with regard to frontal migraine headache. J Plast Reconstr Aesthet Surg. 2017;70:1171–80.
2. Jeon Y, Kim S. Treatment of great auricular neuralgia with real-time ultrasound-guided great auricular nerve block: a case report and review of the literature. Medicine (Baltimore). 2017;96:e6325. https://doi.org/10.1097/MD.0000000000006325.
3. Konschake M, Burger F, Zwierzina M. Peripheral nerve anatomy revisited: modern requirements for neuroimaging and microsurgery. Anat Rec (Hoboken). 2019;302:1325–32.
4. Polacco MA, Butz DR, Bass R, Luu T, Kurum E, DiCarlo A, Maas CS. Nerve blocks prior to microfocused ultrasound treatment are safe and reduce patient discomfort. Aesthet Surg J. 2020;40:887–91.
5. Schoenbrunner A, Konschake M, Zwierzina M, Egro FM, Moriggl B, Janis JE. The great auricular nerve trigger site: anatomy, compression point topography, and treatment options for headache pain. Plast Reconstr Surg. 2022;149:203–11.
6. Stathopoulou TR, Pinelas R, Haar GT, Cornelis I, Viscasillas J. Description of a newapproach for great auricular and auriculotemporal nerve blocks: a cadaveric study in foxes and dogs. Vet Med Sci. 2018;4:91–7.
7. Thallaj A, Marhofer P, Moriggl B, Delvi BM, Kettner SC, Almajed M. Great auricular nerve blockade using high resolution ultrasound: a volunteer study. Anaesthesia. 2010;65:836–40.

# Ultrasound-Guided Cervical Nerve Root Block

Taylan Akkaya, Selin Güven Köse, Mehmet Yılmaz, and Halil Cihan Köse

## Anatomy

The cervical epidural space is bounded anteriorly by the posterior longitudinal ligament and posteriorly by the vertebral laminae and ligamentum flavum. The vertebral pedicles and intervertebral foramen form the lateral borders of the epidural space. The cervical epidural space is approximately 3–4 mm in the C7–T1 range when the cervical spine is flexed [1, 2].

The cervical foramen faces obliquely anteriorly and laterally, with its roof and floor formed by the pedicles of the consecutive vertebrae. Its posterolateral wall is formed largely by the superior articular process of the lower vertebra and partly by the inferior articular process of the upper vertebra and the zygapophysial joint capsule. The anteromedial wall is formed by the lower end of the upper vertebral body, the uncinate process of the lower vertebra, and the posterolateral corner of the intervertebral disc. Immediately lateral to the external opening of the foramen, the vertebral artery emerges just in front of the articular pillars of the zygapophyseal joint [3].

On each side of each cervical spinous process, there are two nerve roots, the ventral root and the dorsal root, which originate from the spinal cord in the vertebral foramen. At typical cervical levels, the ventral and dorsal roots of the spinal nerves continue in the vertebral canal to form the spinal nerve in their respective intervertebral foramen. There are eight cervical spinal nerves, despite only seven cervical vertebrae. The cervical nerve roots exit their respective neural foramina, through the anterior and posterior tubercles of the transverse processes (except for C7, since there is no anterior tubercle at this level), and move anteriorly and inferiorly away from the cervical spine [2]. While the cervical spinal nerve, in its dural sleeve, lies in the lower half of the cervical intervertebral foramen, the epiradicular veins occupy the upper part [3]. The cadaveric image demonstrates the lateral cervical region anatomy at the C 5, 6, and 7 vertebrae level (Fig. 1).

The vertebral, ascending cervical, and deep cervical arteries course close to the cervical spinal nerve roots and often give off branches that contribute to the radicular arteries perfusing the spinal cord. These branches enter the posterior intervertebral foramen through its external opening, which is close to the traditional location of cervical transforaminal epidural injections. In a cadaver study by Huntoon et al. of ten cadavers, it was reported that 20% of branches of the

T. Akkaya
Etlik City Hospital, Department of Anaesthesia and Pain Medicine, Ankara, Turkey

S. G. Köse · H. C. Köse
Kocaeli City Hospital, Department of Pain Medicine, Kocaeli, Turkey

M. Yılmaz (✉)
Ankara University School of Medicine, Department of Anatomy, Ankara, Turkey



T. Akkaya, A. Cömert (eds.), *Practical Guide for Pain Interventions: Head and Neck Sonoanatomy*,
https://doi.org/10.1007/978-3-031-88773-4_9

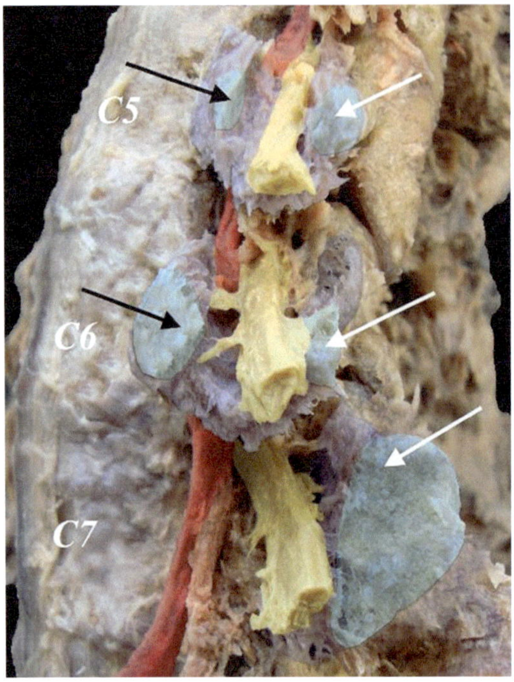


**Fig. 1** Lateral view of cervical spine at C 5, 6, 7 vertebrae levels: purple area is for groove for spinal nerve, blue areas are anterior and posterior tubercles, black arrows indicate anterior tubercle, white arrows indicate posterior tubercle, yellow areas indicate spinal nerves, red region is vertebral artery and C5, C6, C7 indicate vertebral levels

ascending and deep cervical arteries could potentially be punctured within 2 mm of the needle path used in the cervical transforaminal block procedure [4]. These findings suggest that the anatomic location of these arterial branches makes them vulnerable to inadvertent injury or injection, even with correct needle placement.

## Indications

In US-guided CSNRB applications, it is important to determine the target first. In this technique, the target is the nerve root between the anterior and posterior tubercles, especially the ventral ramus. The fluoroscopy-guided technique targets the cervical transforaminal epidural space. It should be clearly stated that in US-guided cervical nerve root injection, the needle targets the extraforaminal area to prevent vascular complications; it would be more appropriate to call it US-guided CSNRB [5].

Since the US-guided CSNRB is applied to the target nerve root without entering the epidural space, it is applied for diagnostic purposes to determine which nerve root is causing the pain. This procedure can also be used to predict the analgesic outcome of cervical discectomy or decompression-fusion surgery. In individuals with persistent radicular pain and nonspecific findings at multiple imaging levels, a CSNRB is used as a diagnostic technique to locate a specific nerve root responsible for the patient's symptoms. Moreover, local anesthetics and steroids administered during these blocks can indirectly reverse the sensitization of spinal sensory neurons observed in chronic pain, allowing patients who have undergone a selective root block to achieve therapeutic results. The amount of local anesthetic to be administered before blockade should be between 0.5 and 1.0 ml, at a concentration that leads to sensory block. This prevents the medication from spreading to the epidural area and nearby tissues, causing false negative or positive reactions. However, if the local anesthetic enters the epidural, subdural, or subarachnoid space, it may block the targeted nerve root as well as cervical nerve roots at other levels and may lose its diagnostic block specific to the targeted nerve root. A reliable response to a CSNRB can accurately determine the level of pathology to be treated, while a negative response to a CSNRB prevents unnecessary spinal surgery. However, missing important details of this technique may lead patients to be referred for other surgeries.

It is also used therapeutically for cervical radicular pain with or without radiculopathy that does not respond to conservative treatment. Cervical radicular pain is characterized by a distribution of pain that resembles the distribution of classical dermatomal maps for cervical nerve roots, although patients may rarely present with pain outside the classical dermatomal distribution. Signs of radiculopathy, such as paresthesia, segmental numbness, weakness, and loss of reflexes, increase the accuracy of the diagnosis. Since cervical radicular pain is frequently caused by foraminal stenosis, the transforaminal approach may maximize the steroid concentration delivered to the affected nerve roots while reducing the required injection volume, and it is effective in the relief of radicular symptoms [5, 6].

## Ultrasound Scan and Technique

Selective nerve root block of the cervical nerve roots is performed using a transforaminal approach. The patient is placed in the lateral decubitus position.

**Step 1: Determination of Cervical Vertebra Level**

A high-resolution linear US probe is placed transverse to the side of the neck to obtain a short-axis view of the spinous process at the cricoid level (Fig. 2). At this level, the probe is moved in a cranial and caudal direction until the cervical tubercles are identified. The US probe may need to be rotated slightly from the transverse position to visualize both tubercles

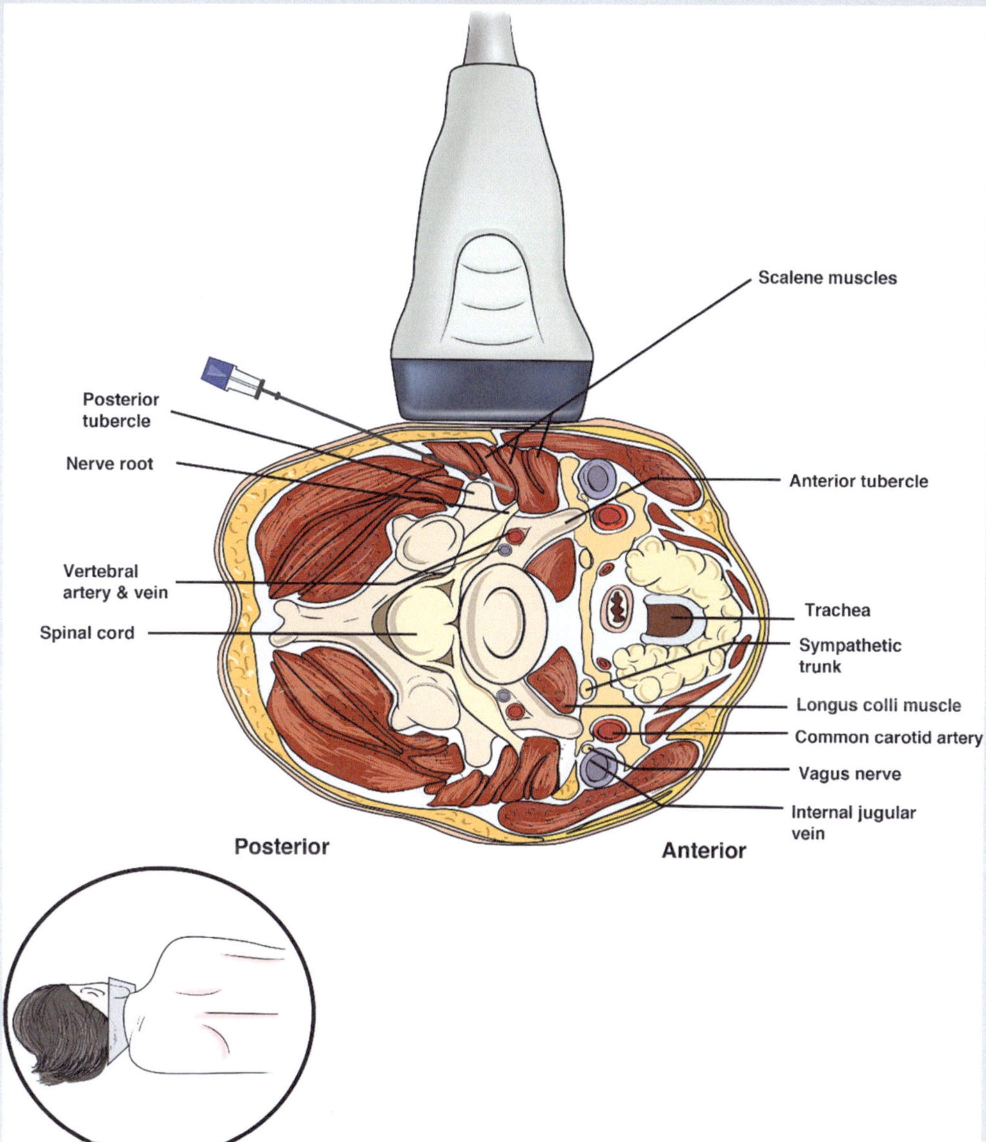


**Fig. 2** Schematic illustration showing the surrounding structures and needle position for ultrasound-guided cervical selective nerve root block at the C6 level

(continued)

because the anterior tubercle is usually slightly cephalic relative to the posterior tubercle. The characteristics of the fifth to seventh cervical vertebrae are important targets for determining cervical vertebral levels.

C5 root block: The cervical fifth level has the same heights of anterior and posterior tubercles, giving it the "2-humped camel" sign. The nerve root emerges from the trough of the transverse process between the tubercles (Fig. 3).

C6 root block: The sixth cervical level has a taller anterior tubercle (known as the Chassaignac's tubercle or the carotid tubercle) but a much shorter posterior tubercle (Fig. 4).

C7 root block: The seventh cervical spinal level can be identified by its unique transverse process with a prominent posterior tubercle but a rudimentary anterior tubercle (Fig. 5). At the C7 level, the C7 nerve root is located just anterior to the posterior tubercle.

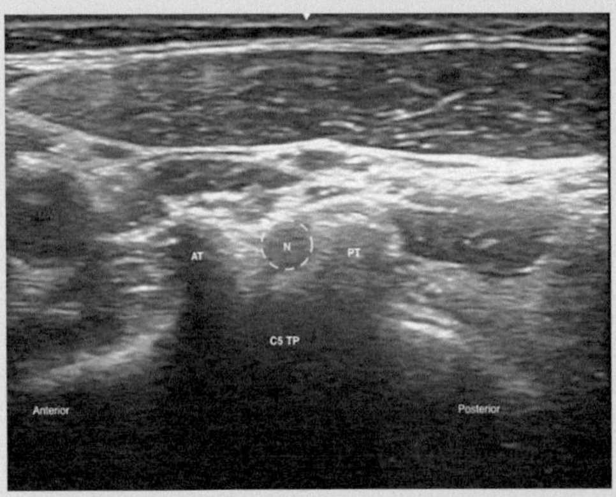


**Fig. 3** Sonographic image showing the anterior tubercle (AT) and the posterior tubercle (PT) of the C5 cervical level (two-humped camel sign). N nerve root, CA carotid artery, TP transverse process

At levels higher than C6, the anterior tubercle shortens and becomes equal to the posterior tubercle, with a narrower space between them than at lower levels [6].

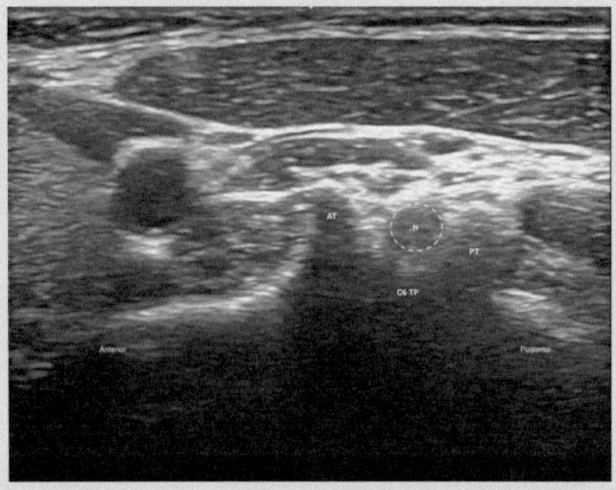


**Fig. 4** Sonographic image showing the taller anterior tubercle (AT) (Chassaignac's tubercle) and the posterior tubercle (PT) of the C6 cervical level. N nerve root, CA carotid artery, TP transverse process

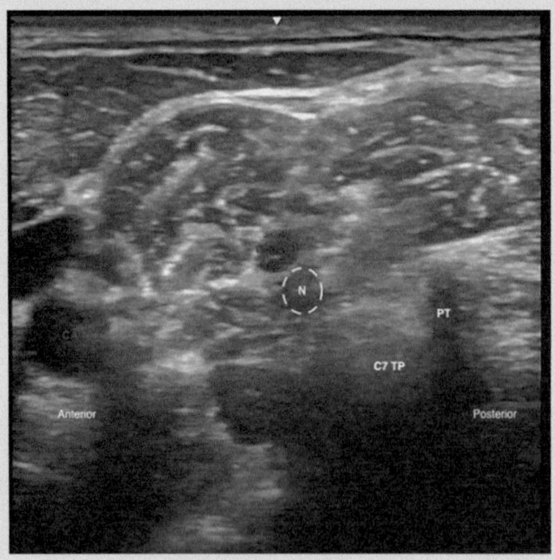


**Fig. 5** Sonographic image showing the posterior tubercle (PT) of the C7 cervical level and vertebral artery (VA). The transverse process of C7 is characterized by the absence of an anterior tubercle. N nerve root, CA carotid artery, TP transverse process

**Step 2: Procedure**

1. Once the cervical vertebrae levels are determined, the US probe can be tilted to clarify the target nerve root.
2. The cervical spinal nerve can be identified in this view between the posterior and anterior tubercles (Fig. 1). At each level, the anterior and posterior tubercle humps will appear as a hyperechoic two-humped camel, with the hypoechoic nerve located between the two humps.
3. When the probe is turned to the longitudinal axis, it is possible to see the entry of the cervical nerve into the foramen and the epidural membrane as a deep hyperechoic line.
4. The probe is returned to the axial position and the spinal nerve here is seen only as a curvature above the cervical foramina.
5. The clinician should apply as little pressure as possible to visualize the pulsation of the vessel near the nerve root.
6. The needle is inserted under real-time US guidance from posterior to anterior using an in-plane technique at a 30-degree angle to the skin to target the corresponding cervical nerve root (from C3 to C8) at the external foraminal opening between the anterior and posterior tubercles of the transverse process. This approach is used because it is less likely to encounter blood vessels behind the nerve root than in front.
7. The target for the tip position is immediately posterior to the emerging nerve root.
8. A color Doppler scan of the injection site is performed to prevent penetration of blood vessels near the nerve root during injection.
9. After negative aspiration to rule out intravascular placement of the needle, the injectate is slowly injected around the nerve root.
10. Drug spread around the cervical nerve can be monitored in real-time. In this stage, intravascular drug spread can also be observed. Failure to visualize the spread of the injected substance around the nerve root during injection may be due to intravascular injection or misdirection of the US probe.
11. The needle is removed, and pressure is applied to the injection site to prevent hematoma formation [7–10].

Recommended Drug Dose:

Diagnostic: 0.5–1 ml bupivacaine 0.25%

Therapeutic: 1–2 ml bupivacaine 0.25% and 4 mg dexamethasone for therapeutic injections

CSNRB can also be performed using fluoroscopy. Especially accurate level determination can be difficult for new practitioners, and level confirmation by fluoroscopy is recommended. It also requires special training and expertise, as visualization of such small vessels (radicular arteries) can be very difficult, especially in obese patients. Real-time fluoroscopy with contrast injection should be used in combination with the US to help identify blood vessels around the foramen.

## Literature Review

### Clinical Practices

Currently, fluoroscopy guidance in oblique view (anterolateral approach) is most commonly used for the cervical transforaminal injection technique [11]. In this technique, the needle is advanced posterior to the intervertebral foramen and anterior to the superior articular process to minimize the risk of vertebral artery or nerve root injury. In addition, different approaches have been described in cervical root block applications, including lateral, posterolateral, and dorsal [12]. Because of the difficulties in the manipulation of the lateral approach, the "modified lateral approach" was developed. This CT-guided approach was applied in 116 cases and was recommended as a reliable approach [13]. In the posterolateral approach described by Kumar et al., the target nerve root was reached by directing the needle into the foramen with a 20–30° oblique angle with C-arm fluoroscopy while the patient was in the lateral position. They described a "safe zone" as the space in the posterosuperior quadrant of the foramen, bounded on the medial side by an imaginary line connecting the midpoints of the articular processes, to minimize the possibility of damage to the dura or blood vessels [14]. In the CT-guided CSNRB using a dorsal approach described by Wolter et al., the mean angle between the needle and the sagittal plane was 26.6° (range, 1–50°) and the mean distance between the needle tip and nerve root was 4.43 mm (range, 0–20 mm) [15]. However, the above methods have poor visualization of blood vessels and nerves, and therefore adverse results including unintended intra-arterial injections resulting in spinal cord injury have been reported, even with strict guidelines. This is where ultrasonography can step in; the US shows not only the target nerves, blood vessels, and surrounding tissues but also the position of the puncture needle, as well as the spread of the injected drug around the nerve in real-time. Hereby, it can have an advantage over fluoroscopy. The US allows vessels to be identified before puncture, whereas fluoroscopy recognizes intravascular injection only after the vessel has been punctured. While fluoroscopy recognizes the intravascular injection only after the blood vessel is punctured, the US allows identification of the blood vessel before puncture. Therefore, the US-guided CSNRB may become a promising modality to replace the fluoroscopic transforaminal approach in clinical practice.

## Cervical Transforaminal Epidural Block Versus CSNRB (Extraforaminal-Periradicular)

In the fluoroscopic approach, the target site is close to the intervertebral foramen in which the procedure is intended to be transforaminal epidural injection. In the US-guided approach, it is critical to determine the target correctly. For CSNRB, the target of the needle is the nerve root in the intertubercular neural groove between the anterior and posterior tubercles of the cervical vertebra outside the foramen, without entering the epidural, subdural, or subarachnoid space. Therefore, CSNRB can also be called extraforaminal or periradicular cervical injection.

In a clinical and cadaveric study, Yamauchi et al. investigated the efficacy and spread of solution in US-guided CNRB. They reported that US-guided CSNRB spreads mainly to the extraforaminal direction and provides adequate analgesic effects for radicular pain by targeting the correct spinal level and vessels [6].

In a randomized study, Jee et al. compared the efficacy and safety of US-guided and fluoroscopy-guided cervical nerve root block. They reported that the US-guided cervical nerve root block produced similar improvement in pain relief, function, and patient satisfaction scores as the fluoroscopy-guided approach without the risk of radiation exposure [16].

Lee et al. compared the technical differences and efficacy between US-guided cervical periradicular steroid injection and traditional fluoroscopy-guided transforaminal epidural injection. Their distance measurements between the two techniques were 1.9–2.3 cm in AP and oblique positions. They showed that US-guided periradicular steroid injection can be an alternative to fluoroscopy-guided transforaminal epidural injection and provide adequate pain relief for the treatment of cervical radicular pain [17].

## Drug Doses

The CSNRB procedure aims to administer the drug to a single nerve root. Although there is no specific standardization, volumes of injectate between 0.5 and 3 ml are used in clinical practice according to the clinical experience of the practitioners. When small volumes are used, the spread may be limited to the targeted nerve root but may be insufficient to block all pain-transmitting fibers. The dural sheath of the spinal nerve is fused to the epineurium at or above the intervertebral foramen. Therefore, when low volumes are used, the anatomical theory is that CSNRB between the anterior and posterior nodes will not result in an unexpected epidural block, whereas when high volumes are used, as in an interlaminar epidural injection technique, the spread of the injectate into the epidural space may result in unintentional blockade of nerve roots at other levels, making the procedure unreliable when used for diagnostic purposes [18].

In a clinical study, Yamauchi demonstrated that real-time US guidance for CSNRB with a total of 2 ml of a mixture of 0.375% ropivacaine and dexamethasone (4 mg) provided a long-term analgesic effect for 1 month in patients despite the absence of intraforaminal epidural spread of the solution. Furthermore, they confirmed the needle-to-nerve root accuracy by fluoroscopy in clinical subjects and dye diffusion followed by dissection in cadavers [6]. Recently, Ma et al. investigated injection spread patterns and therapeutic outcome of US-guided CSNRB with 3 ml injection t (0.33% lidocaine 0.5 ml + compound betamethasone injection 0.5 ml + methylcobalamin injection 1 ml + iohexol 1 ml) in cervical radiculopathy. They reported that the contrast spread into the extraforaminal spaces in 100% (21/21) of the cases, to the foraminal spaces in 61.90% (13/21) of the cases on the postoperative CT scan images, and finally to the epidural spaces in only 2 of 21 cases (9.52%) [18].

## Pulsed Radiofrequency Treatment Combined with Steroid Injection

A neuromodulation technique known as pulsed radiofrequency (PRF) is used to treat the dorsal root ganglion (DRG). The presumed mechanism of action is the stimulation of c-Fos gene expression, which in turn reduces neuronal activity in the dorsal horn and causes sustained pain reduction. Several studies investigated the results of the PRF treatment's neuromodulatory effect on the cervical nerve root. Recently, Chalermkitpanit et al. demonstrated that US-guided periradicular treatment of the cervical nerve root with PRF combined with a steroid injection has a neuromodulatory effect and is considered effective for patients with cervical radicular pain for up to 6 months [19]. In another randomized comparative study, a combination of CSNRB and PRF has been shown to produce better results than CSNRB or PRF alone [20].

## Ultrasound: Advantages and Disadvantages

**Real-Time and Direct Visualization:** The primary advantage of the US technique is the direct observation of soft tissue structures such as blood vessels, nerves, and muscles. US guidance also improves visualization of needle tip placement and distribution of the injectate around the nerves in real time. No vascular injection has been reported in US-guided cervical nerve root injections [5, 16, 18, 21].

**Radiation-Free Imaging:** US guidance can prevent exposure of medical personnel and patients to ionizing radiation. Due to the increased scattered radiation of the C-arm during cervical injections, this is particularly crucial [22].

**Procedure Time:** In a prospective randomized controlled trial, Obernauer et al. examined the procedure time for US-guided versus CT-guided cervical nerve root injections. They found a short procedure time for final needle placement for the US group (2:21 ± 1:43 min) compared to the CT group (10:33 ± 02:30 min) [21].

However, the ultrasonographic technique has its technical limitations. The US cannot visualize the anatomical structure below the bone surface. Therefore, because of the bony artifact of the transverse process, it is not possible to monitor the spread pattern of the high-dose injectate through the foramen into the anterior epidural area and the degree of penetration.

## Complications

Insertion of the needle into the neural foramen and inadvertent injection into the spinal cord may result in quadriplegia or death. The dural puncture may result in sudden total spinal anesthesia associated with loss of consciousness, hypotension, and apnea. If the subdural injection goes unrecognized and epidural doses of local anesthetics are administered, signs and symptoms are similar to those of massive subarachnoid injection with prolonged temporal onset, although the resulting motor and sensory block may be patchy [23].

The cervical epidural space and spinal nerve canals are highly vascular [24]. Injecting local anesthetic directly into an epidural vessel may result in local anesthetic toxicity. The incidence of injection or damage to blood vessels is higher when the C7 nerve root is targeted, as the C7 nerve root runs parallel to the vertebral artery [25].

With proper technique and avoiding excessive sedation, neurologic complications are rare. Although direct trauma to the spinal cord or nerve roots is usually accompanied by pain, some patients may not feel pain. Multiple fluoroscopic views are useful to avoid these complications. If there is significant pain during needle insertion or drug injection, the procedure should be stopped immediately, and the cause of the pain should be determined to avoid the possibility of neural trauma and severe sequelae.

Although not common, infection can occur, especially in patients with cancer-related or acquired immunodeficiency. Early detection and treatment of infection is crucial to avoid potentially life-threatening sequelae. If an epidural abscess occurs, surgical drainage is usually required immediately to prevent spinal cord compression and irreversible neurologic deficits.

Compared to fluoroscopy-guided injection, the US technique offers recognition of periradicular vessels before drug injection and a shorter performance time. However, small vessels are difficult to visualize in the US and require special training and expertise. It is therefore recommended to use real-time fluoroscopy and contrast injection in combination with the US to help identify vessels around the foramen.

Local infection and sepsis due to the potential for hematogenous spread via Batson's plexus, anticoagulant therapy due to the risk of epidural hematoma, and coagulopathy are absolute contraindications for cervical epidural nerve block.

## Recommendations

1. In addition to US confirmation of the needle tip, the use of nerve stimulation will improve the accuracy and safety of CSNRB. The continuous twitch response during the procedure can determine the needle position. The needle tip-nerve distance can be roughly estimated by a stimulating pulse: Over 0.8 mA indicates too far, 0.5–0.8 mA indicates appropriate distance and 0.5 mA or less indicates too close position.
2. Performing therapeutic blocks with non-particulate steroids improves safety.
3. US-guided confirmation with fluoroscopy is recommended before injection into the cervical root. Especially in the identification of blood vessels around the foramen, fluoroscopy-guided injection of radiopaque material is recommended in addition to the US.
4. The vertebral artery usually enters the transverse foramen below C6 in most patients but may be located outside this foramen at the C6 level in up to 10% of patients. Thorough pre-

procedure screening is recommended to identify any abnormal blood vessels near the target nerve root.

5. Aspiration before injection is an unreliable way of detecting intravascular needle placement due to the small size of the vessels in this area. Injection of a test dose of contrast medium is important for the safe performance of the procedure.
6. Any significant pain or sudden increase in resistance during injection indicates needle misplacement, and the practitioner should immediately stop the injection and reassess the position of the needle. Since pain is an important indicator of needle misplacement, excessive patient sedation should be avoided when performing CSNRB.

## References


1. Richardson J, Groen GJ. Applied epidural anatomy. Contin Educ Anaesth Crit Care Pain. 2005;5(3):98–100.
2. Reynolds AF, Roberts PA, Pollay M, et al. Quantitative anatomy of the thoracolumbar epidural space. Neurosurgery. 1985;17:905.
3. Gofur EM, Singh P. Anatomy, back, vertebral canal blood supply. In: StatPearls [Internet]. Treasure Island: Stat Pearls Publishing; 2022. 2023 Jan.
4. Huntoon MA. Anatomy of the cervical intervertebral foramina: vulnerable arteries and ischemic neurologic injuries after transforaminal epidural injections. Pain. 2005;117:104–11.
5. Narouze SN, Vydyanathan A, Kapural L, et al. Ultrasound-guided cervical selective nerve root block: a fluoroscopy-controlled feasibility study. Reg Anesth Pain Med. 2009;34:343–8.
6. Yamauchi M, Suzuki D, Niiya T, Honma H, Tachibana N, Watanabe A, Fujimiya M, Yamakage M. Ultrasound-guided cervical nerve root block: spread of solution and clinical effect. Pain Med. 2011;12:1190–5.
7. Martinoli C, Bianchi S, Santacroce E, Pugliese F, Graif M, Derchi LE. Brachial plexus sonography: a technique for assessing the root level. Am J Roentgenol. 2002;179:699–702.
8. Narouze SN. Ultrasound-guided cervical nerve root block. In: Narouze S, editor. Atlas of ultrasound-guided procedures in interventional pain management. New York: Springer; 2011.
9. Narouze S, Peng P. Ultrasound-guided cervical nerve root block. In: Peng P, Finlayson R, Lee S, Bhatia A, editors. Ultrasound for interventional pain management. Cham: Springer; 2020. https://doi.org/10.1007/978-3-030-18371-4_12.
10. Waldman SD. Cervical selective nerve root block. In: Waldman SD, editor. Atlas of interventional pain management. 4th ed; 2015. https://doi.org/10.1016/B978-0-323-24428-2.00047-4.
11. Schellhas KP, Pollei SR, Johnson BA, Golden MJ, Eklund JA, Pobiel RS. Selective cervical nerve root blockade: experience with a safe and reliable technique using an anterolateral approach for needle placement. AJNR Am J Neurorad. 2007;28:1909–14.
12. Yang D, Xu L, Hu Y, Xu W. Diagnosis and treatment of cervical spondylotic radiculopathy using selective nerve root block (SNRB): where are we now? Pain Ther. 2022;11(2):341–57.
13. Miller TS, Fruauff K, Farinhas J, Pasquale D, Romano C, Schoenfeld AH, Brook A. Lateral decubitus positioning for cervical nerve root block using CT image guidance minimizes effective radiation dose and procedural time. AJNR Am J Neurorad. 2013;34:23–8.
14. Kumar N, Gowda V. Cervical foraminal selective nerve root block: a "two-needle technique" with results. Eur Spine J. 2008;17(4):576–84.
15. Wolter T, Knoeller S, Berlis A, Hader C. CT-guided cervical selective nerve root block with a dorsal approach. AJNR Am J Neuroradiol. 2010;31:1831–6.
16. Jee H, Lee JH, Kim J, Park KD, Lee WY, Park Y. Ultrasound-guided selective nerve root block versus fluoroscopy-guided transforaminal block for the treatment of radicular pain in the lower cervical spine: a randomized, blinded, controlled study. Skeletal Radiol. 2013;42(1):69–78.
17. Lee SH, Kim JM, Chan V, Kim HJ, Kim HI. Ultrasound-guided cervical periradicular steroid injection for cervical radicular pain: relevance of spread pattern and degree of penetration of contrast medium. Pain Med. 2013;14(1):5–13.
18. Ma L, Wang Y, Yao M, Huang B, Deng J, Wen H. Evaluating the extent of ultrasound-guided cervical selective nerve root block in the lower cervical spine: evidence based on computed tomography images. J Pain Res. 2023;16:669–76.
19. Chalermkitpanit P, Pannangpetch P, Kositworakitkun Y, Singhatanadgige W, Yingsakmongkol W, Pasuhirunnikorn P, Tanasansomboon T. Ultrasound-guided pulsed radiofrequency of cervical nerve root for cervical radicular pain: a prospective randomized controlled trial. Spine J. 2023;23(5):651–5.
20. Wang F, Zhou Q, Xiao L, et al. A randomized comparative study of pulsed radiofrequency treatment with or without selective nerve root block for chronic cervical radicular pain. Pain Pract. 2017;17(5):589–95.
21. Obernauer J, GalianoK GH, Bale R, Obwegeser AA, Schatzer R, Loizides A. Ultrasound-guided versus computed tomography-controlled periradicular injections in the middle and lower cervical spine: a prospective randomized clinical trial. Eur Spine J. 2013;22(11):2532–7.

22. Giordano BD, Baumhauer JF, Morgan TL, Rechtine GR. Cervical spine imaging using standard C-arm fluoroscopy: patient and surgeon exposure to ionizing radiation. Spine (Phila Pa 1976). 2008;33(18):1970–6.
23. Wallace MA, Fukui MB, Williams RL, Ku A, Baghai P. Complications of cervical selective nerve root blocks performed with fluoroscopic guidance. AJR Am J Roentgenol. 2007;188(5):1218–21.
24. Flannigan BD, Lufkin RB, McGlade C, Winter J, Batzdorf U, Wilson G, Rauschning W, Bradley WG Jr. MR imaging of the cervical spine: neurovascular anatomy. AJR Am J Roentgenol. 1987;148(4):785–90.
25. Murata S, Iwasaki H, Natsumi Y, Minagawa H, Yamada H. Vascular evaluation around the cervical nerve roots during ultrasound-guided cervical nerve root block. Spine Surg Relat Res. 2019;4(1):18–22.

# Cervical Erector Spinae Block

Hesham Elsharkawy and Ece Yamak Altinpulluk

## Introduction

Erector spinae plane block (ESPB) is a block technique described for the first time by Forero et al. for thoracic neuropathic pain [1]. This technique is performed under ultrasound guidance and involves identifying the transverse process and erector spinae muscle at the level where analgesia is provided and then injecting the local anesthetic underneath the deep fascia of the erector spinae muscle.

ESPB is a technique used not only as a trunk block but also for the upper and lower extremities in multiple indications of acute and chronic pain conditions [2–8].The cervical components of the erector spinae muscle group include longissimus, semispinalis, and iliocostalis cervicis muscles, and they arise from tendons attached to the posterior tubercles of the C2–C7 transverse processes and descend into the thoracic region [1].The prevertebral fascia surrounds the phrenic nerves, brachial plexus, and vertebral column (including the deep cervical muscles of the erector spinae muscle group posteriorly) to form a prevertebral compartment. Therefore, a local anesthetic used in cervical ESP can potentially reach the roots of the brachial plexus within and throughout the prevertebral compartment. Recently, the cervical ESPB has been used for postoperative shoulder pain relief, and it has been shown that the cervical ESP block applied at the C6 and C7 levels can stain the roots of the brachial plexus and dorsal rami [7, 8].

In this chapter, the anatomy of the region, application techniques, indications, contraindications, and complications of cervical ESPB have been discussed to understand its mechanism better.

## Anatomy

### Anatomy of the Cervical Fascia (Concept of Perivertebral Space)

Understanding the detailed anatomy of the fascia in the neck is important for understanding the

H. Elsharkawy (✉)
Department of Anesthesiology, Pain Center, Professor of Anesthesiology, Director of Research, MetroHealth Hospital/Case Western Medical School, Cleveland, OH, USA

Case Western Reserve University, Cleveland, OH, USA

Outcomes Research Consortium, Cleveland, OH, USA

E. Y. Altinpulluk
Morphological Madrid Research Center (MoMaRC), UltraDissection Spain Echo Training School, Madrid, Spain

Member of Outcomes Research Consortium, Cleveland, OH, USA

Board Member of Anesthesiology Clinical Research Office, Ataturk University, Erzurum, Turkey

Faculty of UltraDissection Spain Echo Training School, Madrid, Spain


T. Akkaya, A. Cömert (eds.), *Practical Guide for Pain Interventions: Head and Neck Sonoanatomy*, https://doi.org/10.1007/978-3-031-88773-4_10

mechanism and for the safe performance of the procedure [8].The fascia of the neck can determine the spread pattern of the local anesthetic (LA) in the neck. Concept of perivertebral space: all contents inside the perivertebral fascia can access the LA if the injection is inside that compartment. Those neck compartments act like a conduit for the LA spread to the cervical nerve roots, roots of the brachial plexus, and caudally in the upper thoracic area into the space deep to the erector spinae and rhomboid muscles.

The cervical fascia is anatomically important because it forms concentric layers of the fascia that compartmentalize the neck [9–11]. These fascial layers include the superficial fascia and the deep fascia, with sublayers within the deep fascia [9–11] (Fig. 1).

***Superficial Cervical Fascia*** The superficial cervical fascia covers the subcutaneous layer of the skin in the neck and contains the platysma muscle, cutaneous nerves from the cervical plexus, and superficial vessels and lymph nodes.

***Deep Cervical Fascia*** The deep cervical fascia is deep to the superficial fascia and contains muscles and viscera in compartments to enable structures to slide over each other and to serve as a conduit for neurovascular bundles; it forms the following sublayers: (i) Superficial layer surrounds sternocleidomastoid muscle on the anterior aspect, trapezius muscle posteriorly, and laterally it is roofing the posterior triangle, attached to the tips of the spinous process in the midline. (ii) Deep layer (Perivertebral fascia): The deep layer, named the perivertebral fascia in this book chapter (instead of the prevertebral fascia), as the term "prevertebral fascia" will be used only for the anterior side. It is structured like a tubular sheath around the vertebral column and the deep cervical muscles (cervical erector spinae muscles). The deep muscles of the neck include the longus capitis, the longus colli, and the scalene muscles.

The perivertebral space is defined by the perivertebral fascia, which extends from the cranium base to the coccyx. The perivertebral fascia

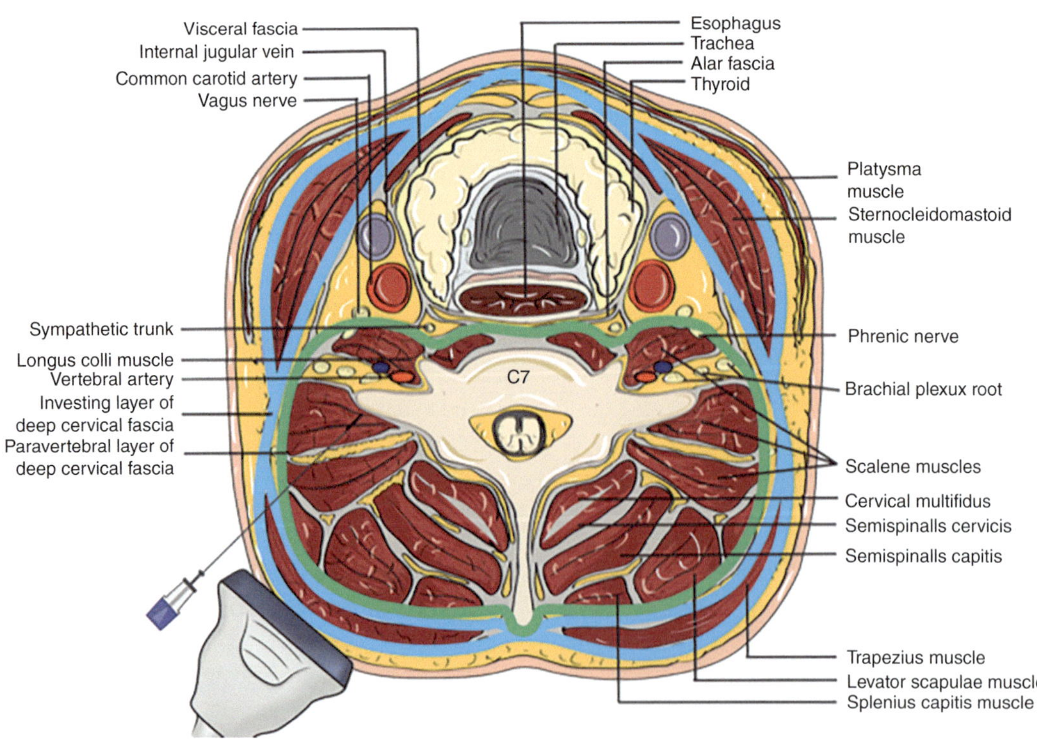


**Fig. 1** Schematic Illustration of Cervical Fascia

accounts for the majority of the deep layer of deep cervical fascia.

***Contents*** Sympathetic trunk, phrenic nerve, brachial plexus, cervical vertebrae, and prevertebral muscles (i.e., longus colli, longus capitis, scalene muscles, levator scapula, and the deep cervical muscles) [1–13].

***Attachments*** Superior attachments are at the skull base. The inferior attachments are continuous with the thoracic cavity, where it is continuous with the thoracolumbar fascia until the coccyx. Posterior attachments are at the spinous processes of cervical and thoracic vertebrae. Lateral attachments are transverse processes (TP) of cervical and thoracic vertebrae.

***Boundaries*** Perivertebral space; the prevertebral fascia forms a complete border around the perivertebral space. It arches in front of the vertebral bodies from transverse processes on either side to define the anterior, prevertebral portion of the perivertebral space, which contains the roots of the brachial plexus and extends posteriorly from transverse processes on either side to the midline, where it fuses with the nuchal ligament to define the posterior, paraspinal portion of the perivertebral space. This is particularly important as this fascial sheath creates a potential cervical space for the spread of LA.

***Anatomy of the Muscles of the Neck*** The muscles of the neck are organized and grouped with the cervical fascia. The platysma muscle is within the superficial fascia. The sternocleidomastoid, trapezius, and the prevertebral muscles are within the deep investing fascia (perivertebral fascia).

The perivertebral muscles are located between the prevertebral fascia and the cervical vertebrae. Longus colli and capitis muscles are located superiorly between the anterior side of the base of the skull and inferiorly between the cervical and upper thoracic vertebrae.

Scalene muscles are classified into three groups (anterior, middle, and posterior scalenes). They attach between cervical transverse processes and ribs 1 and 2. The neurovascular structures are between the middle layer (middle scalene) and the deep layer (anterior scalene). Then, both the cervical and brachial plexuses way out from the vertebral column between the anterior and middle scalenes [9–19]. (Fig. 1).

## Injection Technique

The procedure can be performed in the prone or lateral decubitus position. A high-frequency (12–15 MHz) linear-array transducer is placed in a transverse orientation lateral to the posterior midline. It can be done at any level according to the indications, but it has been described in the literature at the C6 and C7 levels [7].

For the C6 injection, the transducer is placed in transverse orientation at the C6 TP level, which is identified as the Chassaignac tubercle (anterior tubercle of the transverse process of C6). Then the erector spinae plane between the tip of the posterior tubercle of the C6 TP and the overlying erector spinae muscle is identified. For the C7 injection, the transducer is placed in transverse orientation at the C7 TP, which is identified by the prominent posterior tubercle and absent anterior tubercle. The erector spinae plane is located between the tip of the C7 TP and the overlying erector spinae muscle. The needle is inserted in the posterior-anterior direction through the trapezius and levator scapulae muscles until it contacts the posterior tip of the TP. The correct needle tip position is confirmed by hydrodissection using 2–3 ml of saline to separate the erector spinae muscles from the TP (Figs. 2 and 3).

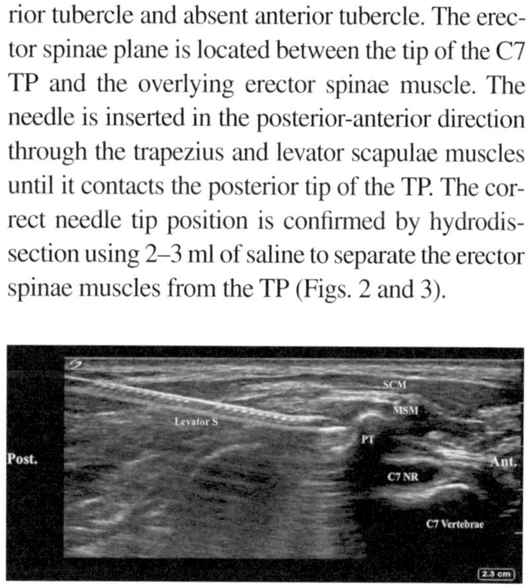


**Fig. 2** Ultrasound image of The Cervical Erector Spinae Block on a cadaver model. SCM Sternocleidomastoid muscle, MSM Middle Scalene Muscle, C7 NR Cervical 7 nerve root, PT Posterior Tubercle, Levator S Levator Scapula Muscle

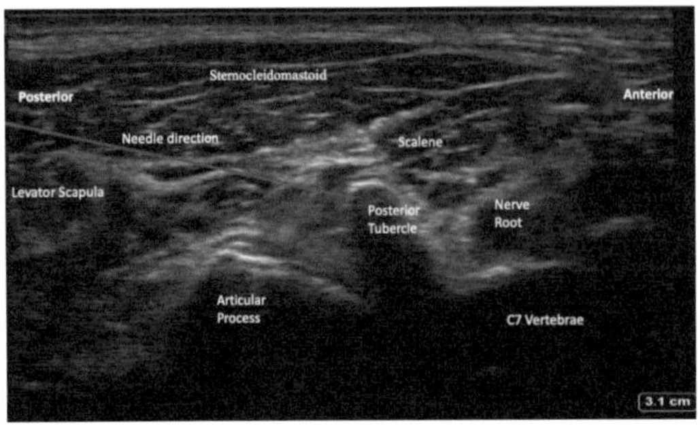


**Fig. 3** Ultrasound image of The Cervical Erector Spinae Block at level C7

## Indications

This block can be considered as an alternative to the interscalene brachial plexus block, cervical dorsal medial nerve branch blocks, and occipital nerve blocks and can be used in the following indications.

- Postoperative shoulder analgesia
- Shoulder disarticulation
- Shoulder arthroscopy
- Scapular fracture analgesia and postoperative pain
- Cervical spine surgery, posterior fusion instrumentation
- Posterior atlantoaxial fusion surgery
- Cervical spondylosis, facet arthropathy
- Occipital pain and headaches
- Myofascial pain in the upper thoracic and cervical area

## Contraindications

Standard contraindications apply to ESPB as well, and absolute contraindications include local infection, allergy to local anesthetics, and a known bleeding diathesis due to its deep block nature. Hemodynamic instability, known neurological disorders, and anatomical abnormalities can be considered relative contraindications. Kwon et al. emphasized the need for caution regarding phrenic nerve paralysis, especially when cervical ESPB is used bilaterally for cervical posterior neck surgeries [20].

## Dose and Volume of Local Anesthetic

Since this is a plane block, it is volume-dependent, and the affected segment area may vary according to the volume doses applied. Generally, a 0.2 ml/kg local anesthetic dose (20 ml) provides an adequate block in unilateral blocks [21]. The dose of local anesthetic needs to be considered for the size of the patient to ensure the maximum safe dose is not exceeded, especially with bilateral blocks. Randomized controlled studies are needed in terms of optimal local anesthetic dose and efficacy.

## Mechanism of Action

Elsharkawy et al. have demonstrated that injection at the C6 and C7 levels consistently distributes to the roots of the brachial plexus anteriorly in addition to relevant nerves, including the long thoracic, dorsal scapular, and suprascapular nerves [9]. Moreover, injectate craniocaudal spread has shown that injection at both C6 and C7 levels spreads similarly to cover the target sensory level of C5–C8 and also the dorsal cervical rami of the involved segments. Therefore, this has been clarified and explained how the cervical ESP block can provide analgesia in patients undergoing major shoulder surgery and cervical spine surgery.

## Advantages

Bony contact all the time at either C6 or C7 may decrease the risk of vertebral artery injury because there is no direct contact between the nerve roots with the needle and a major vessel in the track of the needle, and it can be done under general anesthesia. It can cover more than the roots of the brachial plexus, T1, T2, and T3, as they are spread deep to the rhomboid intercostals; it may cover the upper chest, and block the suprascapular nerve. It can potentially cover the cervical plexus, branches from C2 to C4 (lesser occipital (C2, C3), great auricular (C2, C3), transverse cervical (C2, C3), and supraclavicular nerves (C3, C4); these initially run posteriorly and soon pierce the prevertebral fascia). Potentially this technique can be used as an alternative If the inter-scalene location is not possible technically due to disarticulation, the presence of central line or pacemaker wires, or in patients with difficult anatomy.

The skin overlying the clavicle is innervated by the supraclavicular branches of the superficial cervical plexus. Clavicular bony pain requires a combination of superficial cervical plexus block with interscalene brachial plexus block (that can be targeted toward C5/6 roots higher in the interscalene groove). Cervical ESPB theoretically can block those nerves.

## Limitations

Most of the evidence of the mechanism of action has been made using cadaveric studies along with limitations of cadaver studies, and there are anatomical and physiological differences between living and deceased tissues. Therefore, it is challenging to assess the difficulty of the procedure and assume the mechanism of action. This approach has the possibility of epidural or subarachnoid spread of local anesthetic if the needle advances beyond the transverse process. Vertebral artery injury also is possible, especially with the C7 injection, but those complications also have been reported with the classical interscalene approach. Cervical ESPB could potentially lead to phrenic nerve block as LA can spread to the roots of the phrenic nerve and/or the nerve anterior to the anterior scalene muscle, particularly with larger volumes of LA [20]. In addition, it potentially can block the recurrent laryngeal nerve. Future studies are needed to study the safety profile of the cervical ESB versus interscalene and compare it with T 2–3 ESPB.

There is some similarity between the current technique and the deep cervical plexus block. The C6–C7 ESPB is injected inside the perivertebral fascia and posterior to the transverse process at C6 and C7 levels, controversially at C3--4 levels around the nerve roots for the deep cervical plexus block.

## Complications

Although cervical ESPB has a motor-sparing effect, high-volume LA can potentially spread to the cervical epidural space, and therefore hypotension, prolonged motor block, upper extremity weakness, delayed mobilization, and delayed hospital discharge may occur. Although the cervical ESPB target injection site is far from the phrenic nerve, cervical nerves, and sympathetic nerves, the cadaver studies showed that LA might spread to the phrenic nerve, so it is necessary to be cautious when performing bilateral ESPB in the cervical posterior neck surgery [9, 20, 21]. Local anesthesia toxicity is always a potential risk due to the use of high doses and volume of local anesthetic and the vascular structures in the region. Although no cases have been reported before, basic monitoring should be done, and resuscitation equipment should be ready.

## Needle Trauma

Although bone tissue is targeted, there is a risk of direct needle trauma since the procedure is performed in areas close to the cervical roots and vertebral artery. The risks of bleeding complications are not yet known. There is no evidence for the stratification of the risk of bleeding, but the recommendation is that the American Society of Regional Anesthesia and Pain Medicine guidelines for deep peripheral blocks be followed due to vascular structures in the block area.

## Evidence and Discussion

No randomized controlled studies have been found related to cervical ESPB. The cervical fascia is the main fascia of the neck and has different layers [9–11]. The superficial cervical fascia is a subcutaneous layer of the skin in the neck and contains the platysma muscle, cutaneous nerves from the cervical plexus, and superficial vessels and lymph nodes. The deep cervical fascia consists of three layers—“investing,” “pretracheal,” and “prevertebral” layers—which are also known

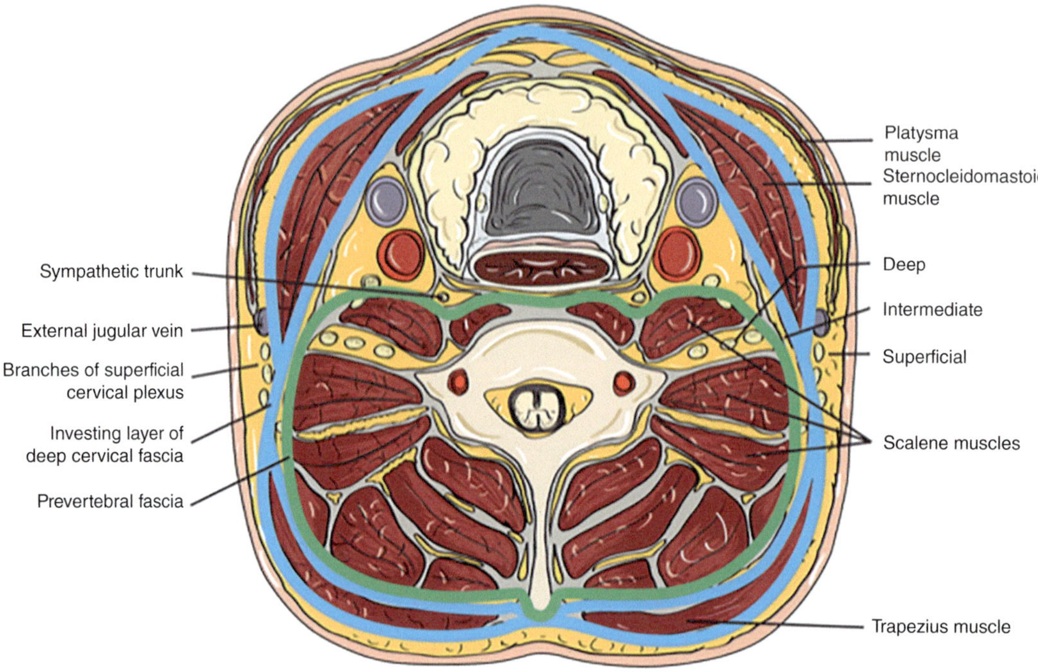


**Fig. 4** Schematic Illustration of Cervical Fascia

as the superficial, middle, and deep layers, respectively (Fig. Fig. 4) [9–11]. Deep investing fascia contains trapezius and sternocleidomastoid muscles. This fascia composes the roof of the posterior triangle between the trapezius and sternocleidomastoid muscles and attaches to the posterior aspects of the spinous processes at the midline. The pretracheal (middle) layer of fascia is situated in the anterior neck and covers the hyoid bone superiorly and the thorax inferiorly. The prevertebral (deep) layer is one of the major clinically relevant structures in the cervical ESP block. This layer attaches to the ligamentum nuchae and fully encircles the vertebrae, scalene, erector spinae, and associated vertebrae muscles, as well as neurological structures such as the cervical portion of the sympathetic trunk ganglia, phrenic nerve, brachial plexus, and the nerves to the rhomboids and serratus anterior. Thus, any injections under the prevertebral layer may allow the potential spread to its enclosed structures.

The cervical ESPB is performed with a more posterior approach than the cervical paravertebral block. Instead of the needle being "walked off" the bony cervical TP, the roots of the brachial plexus, the ESPB injection is performed posterior to the cervical TP. In the cervical ESPB, the needle tip should be all the time in contact with the TP [9]. Although the placement of the needle seems relatively safe since ESPB is made by targeting the posterior end of the TP posterior tubercle, away from structures such as the phrenic nerve, cervical nerves, and sympathetic nerves, it has been seen in the case series that there is a risk of phrenic nerve paralysis [21]. However, it can be said that this needle placement is further away from the phrenic nerve compared to the interscalene block and that TP, which is the bone structure in front of the needle tip, can protect the vertebral artery [9, 21]. Ultrasound-guided cervical (C6 and C7) ESP injections consistently in cadaver studies stain the roots of the brachial plexus and dorsal rami. This study may support the concept that the cervical ESP block has the potential to provide analgesia for patients undergoing shoulder and cervical spine surgeries [9].

Cervical ESPB can be an alternative option to brachial plexus block/ or blocking the terminal branches like suprascapular and axillary nerves.

Cervical ESP does not eliminate the phrenic nerve involvement but theoretically decreases this side effect compared to the classical brachial plexus block.

In recent years, at the cervical region, new paraspinal interfacial blocks (PIP) such as multifidus cervicis plan block (MCPB), retrolaminar, and inter-semispinalis block (ISP) have been developed. These blocks have been shown to block the dorsal cervical nerves without needle entry into the paravertebral space [22–25]. All these interfascial plane blocks have been seen as promising alternatives to neural axial blockade for various procedures. In contrast to paravertebral blocks, it can be theoretically said that the injection site is simpler and safer as it is far from the neural axis. These blocks target the dorsal rami, not the ventral rami; therefore, ESPB has been excluded from the paraspinal interfascial block category in the study by Xu et al. [26]. Ohgoshi has claimed that in the case of cervical spine surgery, PIP blocks are preferred to cervical ESPB as they only block the posterior spinal nerve [27]. Also, it has been claimed that it provides cervical brachial plexus block in ESPB, whereas the anatomical boundary defining local diffusion of local anesthesia in MCP and ISP blocks is the semispinalis cervicis muscle. According to Tsui and Elsharkawy, the anatomical barrier to local anesthetic distribution is not the semispinalis cervicis muscle but the individual anatomical disposition of the patient's neck fascia [28]. In addition, they stated that when higher volume LA is used, LA spreads over a wide area, regardless of the type of PIP block. In PIP blocks, the injection point is more posterior between the different muscles of the cervical ESP group, far from the ventral rami and the phrenic nerve. Although the risk of phrenic involvement is less in blocks targeting the dorsal rami, it is still theoretically possible since it is the injection into that compartment. The volume is a key factor for the chances of the LA spreading to the phrenic nerve. PIP blocks can be relatively difficult to implement, as they are blocks made between muscles in the facial planes without bony markings that complicate the separation of the different layers.

Preventing phrenic nerve involvement while performing ESPB block; the other technique described is the cranial directing of the ESP catheter placed at the T2 level, followed by slow titration of the LA. This may be an easier and safer option to prevent or reduce phrenic nerve involvement.

## Cervical Erector Spinae Peripheral Nerve Catheter and Peripheral Nerve Stimulator Implant

A continuous technique and implantation of a peripheral nerve stimulator (unpublished data, 2022) can be successfully used for many indications, including chronic postoperative pain conditions after cervical fusion surgery. A 17- or 18-gauge Tuohy needle can be used for catheter placement. The needle is inserted through the trapezius, levator scapulae, and deep cervical muscles (i.e., erector spinae muscles) until it contacts the posterior tubercle of the C7 transverse process [4]. After a negative aspiration is confirmed, 1–3 ml of local anesthetic is injected slowly to confirm penetration of the appropriate fascial layers. A total of 10 ml of the same solution is then injected slowly; a catheter is subsequently advanced 2–4 cm past the tip of the needle. For continuous infusions, ropivacaine at concentrations of 0.1–0.2% is used with a basal infusion rate of 6–8 ml an hour and a patient-controlled bolus of 5–12 ml every hour.

## Cervical Erector Spinae Block in the Anticoagulated Patient

The risks of bleeding complications are unknown, and there are no specific recommendations, but the American Society of Regional Anesthesia and Pain Medicine guidelines for deep peripheral blocks should be considered in patients on anticoagulants who are receiving ESPB. Risk versus benefits should be carefully considered.

## Future Research

Further clinical studies are needed to compare interscalene and ESPB regarding the safety and efficacy of cervical ESP block. In addition, studies are needed to investigate the craniocaudal dermatomal spread of the block, optimal LA dosage, and the incidence of phrenic nerve involvement.

## Conclusion

Current evidence illustrates that cervical ESP injections resulted in the involvement of the ventral rami of C5 to C7 (i.e., brachial plexus), less incidence of phrenic nerve involvement also consistently spread to the posterior aspect of the erector spinae muscles, and the dorsal rami.

## References


1. Forero M, Adhikary SD, Lopez H, Tsui C, Chin KJ. The erector spinae plane block: a novel analgesic technique in thoracic neuropathic pain. Reg Anesth Pain Med. 2016;41:621–7.
2. Chung K, Kim ED. Continuous erector spinae plane block at the lower lumbar level in a lower extremity complex regional pain syndrome patient. J Clin Anesth. 2018;48:30–1.
3. Bang S, Choi J, Kim ED. A high thoracic erector spinae plane block is used for sympathetic block in patients with upper extremity complex regional pain syndrome. J Clin Anesth. 2020;60:99–100.
4. Hamadnalla H, Elsharkawy H, Shimada T, Maheshwari K, Esa WA, Tsui BC. Cervical erector spinae plane block catheter for shoulder disarticulation surgery. Can J Anesth. 2019;66:1129–31.
5. Forero M, Rajarathinam M, Adhikary SD, Chin KJ. Erector spinae plane block for the management of chronic shoulder pain: a case report. Can J Anaesth. 2018;65:288–93.
6. Tsui BCH, Mohler D, Caruso TJ, et al. Cervical erector spinae plane block catheter using a thoracic approach: an alternative to brachial plexus blockade for forequarter amputation. Can J Anaesth. 2019;66:119–20.
7. Feigl G, Hammer GP, Litz R, et al. The intercarotid or alar fascia, other cervical fascias, and their adjacent spaces – a plea for clarification of cervical fascia and spaces terminology. J Anat. 2020;237(1):197–207. https://doi.org/10.1111/joa.13175.
8. Hamadnalla H, Elsharkawy H, Shimada T, et al. Cervical erector spinae plane block catheter for shoulder disarticulation surgery. Can J Anaesth. 2019;66:1129–31.
9. Elsharkawy H, Ince I, Hamadnalla H, Drake RL, Tsui BCH. Cervical erector spinae plane block: a cadaver study. Reg Anesth Pain Med. 2020;45:552–6.
10. Stecco A, Meneghini A, Stern R, Stecco C, Imamura M. Ultrasonography in myofascial neck pain: randomized clinical trial for diagnosis and follow-up. Surg Radiol Anat. 2014;36:243–53.
11. Tschopp KP, Gysin C. Local injection therapy in 107 patients with myofascial pain syndrome of the head and neck. ORL J Otorhinolaryngol Relat Spec. 1996;58:306–10.
12. Netter FH. Atlas of human anatomy. 6th ed. Philadelphia: Elsevier; 2014. PA: Churchill Livingstone: Elsevier
13. Chapter 43. Susan standring gray's anatomy. Elsevier Limited; 2016. p. 709–750.e2.
14. Morton D, Albertine K, Foreman B. The big picture: gross anatomy. New York: The McGraw-Hill Companies Inc.; 2011.
15. Morton DA, Foreman KB, Albertine KH. The big picture: gross anatomy. 2nd ed. New York: McGraw-Hill; 2018. p. 1. Online resource.
16. Moore K, Dalley AF, Agur AM. Clinically oriented anatomy. 7th ed. Baltimore: Lippincott Williams & Wilkins; 2014. p. 988.
17. Zhang MN, Nicholson H, Nash L. Investing layer of the cervical fascia of the neck may not exit. Anesthesiology. 2006;104:1344–5.
18. Pandit JJ, Dorje P, Satya-Krishna R. Investing layer of the cervical fascia of the neck may not exist. Anesthesiology. 2006;104:1344.
19. Natale G, Condino S, Stecco A, Soldani P, Belmonte MM, Gesi M. Is the cervical fascia an anatomical proteus? Surg Radiol Anat. 2015;37:1119–27.
20. Kwon AH, Xu JL. Cervical erector spinae plane block: is it feasible for cervical spine surgeries? Reg Anesth Pain Med. 2021;46:552–3.
21. Ma D, Wang R, Wen H, Li H, Jiang J. Cervical erector spinae plane block as a perioperative analgesia method for shoulder arthroscopy: a case series. J Anesth. 2021;35:446–50.
22. Ueshima H, Otake H. RETRACTED: blocking of multiple posterior branches of cervical nerves using a cervical interfascial plane block. J Clin Anesth. 2017;38:5.
23. Ohgoshi Y, Izawa H, Kori S, Matsukawa M. Multifidus cervicis plane block is effective for cervical spine surgery. Can J Anesth. 2017;64:329–30.
24. Ohgoshi Y, Nishizakura R, Takahashi Y, Takeda K, Nakayama H, Kawamata M, Kurahashi K. Novel ultrasound-guided inter-Semispinal plane block: a comparative pilot study in healthy volunteers. J Anesth. 2018;32:143–6.
25. Hochberg U, de Santiago MJ. Ultrasound-guided retrolaminar cervical block. Reg Anesth Pain Med. 2022;47:73–4.

26. Xu JL, Tseng V. Proposal to standardize the nomenclature for paraspinal interfascial plane blocks. Reg Anesth Pain Med. 2019;44:1106–7.
27. Ohgoshi Y. Semispinalis capitis muscle is a key factor in defining cervical nerve block effect. Reg Anesth Pain Med. 2021;46:457–8.
28. Tsui BCH, Elsharkawy H. Novel cervical erector spinae plane block: interfacial layers remain important in the spread of anesthetics. Reg Anesth Pain Med. 2021;46:458–9.

# Cervical Plexus Block

Ece Yamak Altinpulluk and Mario Fajardo Perez

## Introduction

The cervical plexus (CP) block provides analgesia and anesthesia for the neck and head region [1]. Its most common clinical use is carotid endarterectomy. Other procedures performed using CP block are procedures in the neck area, such as superficial neck procedures, analgesia for clavicle fractures, thyroid surgery, and ear surgery [2–9]. Conventionally, CP blocks were categorized as superficial or deep; however, in 2004, Telford and Stoneham [10] recommended the intermediate CP block involving a sub-investing layer of the deep cervical fascia injection based on the cadaveric study by Pandit et al. [11].

Choquet et al. improved the definition of intermediate CP blocks using the ultrasound technique in 2010 [12]. With the development of technology and the widespread ultrasound use in the head/neck region, the CP block has begun to be applied more safely and accurately by simply identifying landmarks such as muscles and cervical vertebrae under ultrasound guidance [13]. This chapter addresses the anatomy of the cervical plexus, indications for the blocks, and ultrasound-guided techniques. Also, the complications associated with the CP block and how they should be managed have been highlighted.

## Anatomy

### Cervical Fascia

Fascia is a connective tissue surrounding structures within the body. Fascia (a) stabilizes and separates the muscles from other internal organs, (b) forms compartments, (c) is a storage medium for fat and water, (d) passage for nerves, vessels, and lymph. There are three types of fascia such as superficial, deep, and visceral fascia. Cervical fascia is anatomically important because it forms concentric layers of the fascia that compartmentalize the neck. Therefore, cervical fascial variation may play an important act in the pathogenesis of chronic neck pain, understanding surgical orientation, and the spread of disease (cancer, infection, etc.). The cervical fascia is the main fascia of the neck and has different layers [14, 15].

E. Y. Altinpulluk
Morphological Madrid Research Center (MoMaRC), UltraDissection Spain Echo Training School, Madrid, Spain

Member of Outcomes Research Consortium, Cleveland, OH, USA

Board Member of Anesthesiology Clinical Research Office, Ataturk University, Erzurum, Turkey

Faculty of UltraDissection Spain Echo Training School, Madrid, Spain

M. F. Perez (✉)
CEO of MoMaRC and Ultra Dissection Spain Echo Training School, Madrid, Spain



T. Akkaya, A. Cömert (eds.), *Practical Guide for Pain Interventions: Head and Neck Sonoanatomy*,
https://doi.org/10.1007/978-3-031-88773-4_11

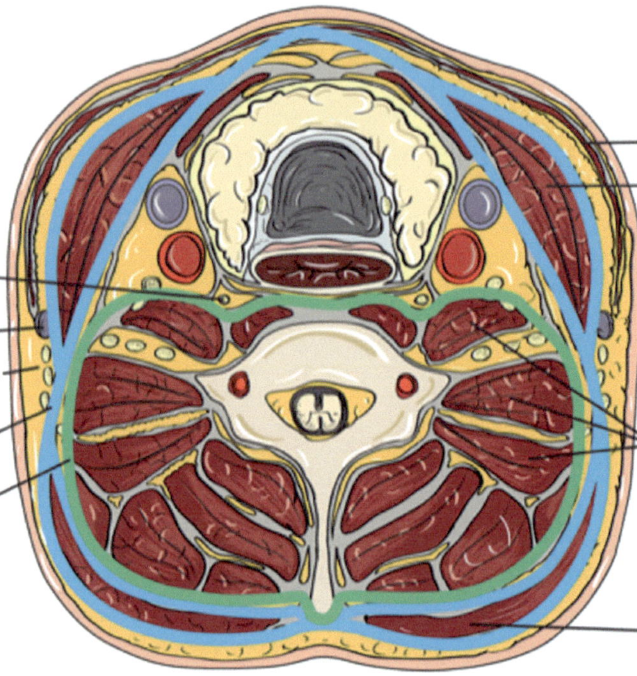


**Fig. 1** Schematic illustration of the cervical fascia

The superficial fascia layer of the cervical fascia covers the surface of the neck and contains platysma muscle, cutaneous veins, arteries, nerves, and branches from the cervical plexus. The deep fascia has compartments for muscles, vessels, and viscera. Subdivisions of the deep fascia include deep investing fascia, pretracheal fascia, prevertebral fascia, and carotid sheath (Fig. 1). Deep investing fascia contains trapezius and sternocleidomastoid muscles. This fascia is composed of the roof of the posterior triangle between the trapezius and sternocleidomastoid muscles. The investing layer of deep fascia is pierced by the cutaneous branches of the cervical plexus and external jugular vein. The boundaries of this fascia are hyoid, mandible, and sternum on the front; clavicula and scapula on the side; occipital bone nuchal ligament, and trapezius along the back [16, 17].

The other fascial component is the pretracheal fascia. This part forms a visceral component and includes the thyroid, trachea, esophagus, recurrent laryngeal nerve, and parathyroid glands. The posterior prethracheal fascia border has a specific name which is called buccopharyngeal fascia. Between these two fascial planes, the pharynx goes up higher, and the esophagus goes down. The other fascia is the prevertebral fascia (muscular component). This fascial plane includes the vertebral colon. There are longus colli muscles, longus capitis muscles, scalene muscles (anterior, middle, and posterior), levator scapulae muscles, and paraspinal muscles in this fascial plane. The sympathetic trunk is not in this fascial plane. The phrenic nerve is in the front of the anterior scalene muscle. The cervical/brachial plexus is between the anterior and middle scalene muscles. Prevertebral fascia forms an axillary sheath that envelops the brachial plexus, subclavian, and axillary artery. Prevertebral fascia has a subdivision on the front, which is called alar fascia. Therefore, the prevertebral fascia has two layers on the front. Alar fascia fuses with buccopharyngeal fascia between the T1 and T4 vertebral level. The carotid sheath (vascular component includes internal jugular vein, carotid arteries, and nervous vagus) is formed by adjacent facial sleeves (deep investing fascia, prethracheal fascia, and prevertebral fascia). The carotid sheath has ansacervicalis within the wall. Additionally, if clinicians do not reach a consensus on which fascia the infrahyoid muscles are in, we can say that these muscles are located within the deep cervical fascia [16, 17].

## Anatomical Spaces

Fascial layers in the neck define some potential spaces. In healthy patients, these anatomical spaces are closed. However, some conditions like infection can widen these spaces. One of these spaces is the retropharyngeal fascia; this is the space between the alar fascia and buccopharyngeal fascia. The other space is the danger space, between the alar fascia and prevertebral fascia. If infection occurs in the retropharyngeal fascia, this may bulge anteriorly and restrict breathing and swallowing. The infection could spread to mediastinum, if not to the fusion, between the alar fascia and buccopharyngeal fascia. However, in the danger space, the infection can spread from the skull base to the mediastinum. Although there are many different opinions, it should not be forgotten that the alar fascia collapses in healthy patients, so only the retropharyngeal fascia is mentioned [1, 16, 17].

## Triangles of the Neck

The triangles of the neck are the regions of the neck bounded by the muscles. Knowing and identifying the triangles is important because they facilitate the description of the neck anatomy and help to identify structures such as glands, nerves, vessels, and lymph nodes. When the block has performed this triangle, a landmark helps to identify smaller landmarks within. The sternocleidomastoid muscle (SCM) is a guide for the identification of the neck because it divides the neck into two major neck triangles: the anterior and the posterior triangle of the neck. The anterior triangle (AT) of the neck is subdivided into four smaller triangles, and the posterior triangle (PT) is divided into two smaller triangles.

AT of the neck's borders consists of the SCM, mandible, and anterior midline of the neck. AT is subdivided into four triangles as submental, carotid, submandibular, and muscular triangles. The submandibular triangle is between the anterior and posterior belly of the digastric muscle as well as the mandible, and it includes the facial vessels, lingual vessels, the submandibular gland and lymph nodes (anteriorly), submental vessels, caudal part of the parotid gland (posteriorly), mylohyoid, and hypoglossal (CN XII) nerve. The submental triangle is bordered by the mandible, the anterior belly of the digastric muscle, and the hyoid bone. This triangle includes the anterior jugular vein and submental lymph nodes. Carotid triangle borders consist of the posterior belly of the digastric muscle, the superior belly of the omohyoid muscle, and SCM. It includes arteries such as common carotid, external carotid, internal carotid artery, veins such as common facial, internal jugular, lingual, middle thyroid veins, superior thyroid and nerves such as hypoglossal nerve (CN XII), vagus nerve (CN X), part of the sympathetic trunk, ansacervicalis and branches from cervical plexus. The muscular triangle is bordered by the omohyoid, sternohyoid, and SCM and includes anterior jugular veins, superior and inferior thyroid arteries, thyroid gland, parathyroid glands, trachea, larynx, and esophagus.

The posterior triangle is the area between SCM, trapezius, and the middle one-third of the clavicula. The roof of the posterior triangle is the deep investing fascia, and the floor of it is the prevertebral fascia (Figs. 1 and 2).

Contents of the posterior triangle, which pierces deep investing fascia, are cutaneous nerves from the cervical plexus and external jugular vein. There is the omohyoid muscle at the floor of the PT and it divides the PT into an occipital triangle, which includes the accessory nerve (CN XI), branches of the cervical plexus, supraclavicular nerve, the uppermost part of the brachial plexus, and a supraclavicular triangle, which includes the third part of the subclavian artery, nerve to subclavius muscle, lymph nodes, and brachial plexus trunks. If the prevertebral fascia is removed, splenius capitis, levator scapulae, and all scalene muscles are seen. Additionally, the brachial plexus (C5–T1) is placed between the middle and anterior scalene muscles. Also, the subclavian artery and vein are placed in that area [16, 17].

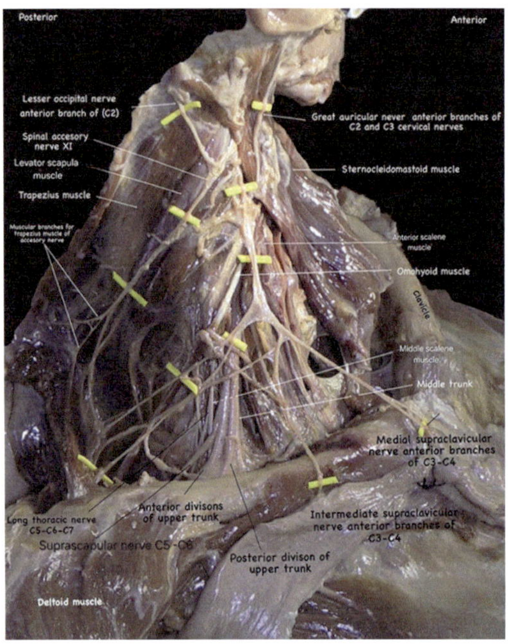


**Fig. 2** Cervical plexus branches on cadaveric model

## Cervical Plexus

The cervical plexus is the cluster of nerves formed by the ventral rami from the first four spinal nerves (C1–C4). CP consists of two nerve branches: muscular (deep) branches and cutaneous (superficial branches). The cervical plexus nerves pass from medial to lateral under the sternocleidomastoid muscle and pierce the superficial cervical fascia at the lateral margin corresponding to the Erb point. Cutaneous branches of the CP provide sensory innervation of the skin of the anterolateral neck. These are the supraclavicular nerve (C3, C4), the greater auricular nerve (C2, C3), the transverse cervical nerve (C2, C3), and the lesser occipital nerve (C2, C3) [1] (Figs. 2 and 3).

The muscular branches of the CP are branches from the ansacervicalis and the phrenic nerve. Fibers arising anteromedially from the upper (C1–C2) and lower (C2–C3) roots converge at the level of the omohyoid central tendon to form a loop called ansacervicalis. The phrenic nerve (primarily from C4 and from C3 to C5) innervates the diaphragm and pericardium and ansa cervicalis supplies motor branches to the infrahyoid muscles and SCM. Additionally, the cervical

**Fig. 3** Schematic illustration of the superficial cutaneous branches of the cervical plexus

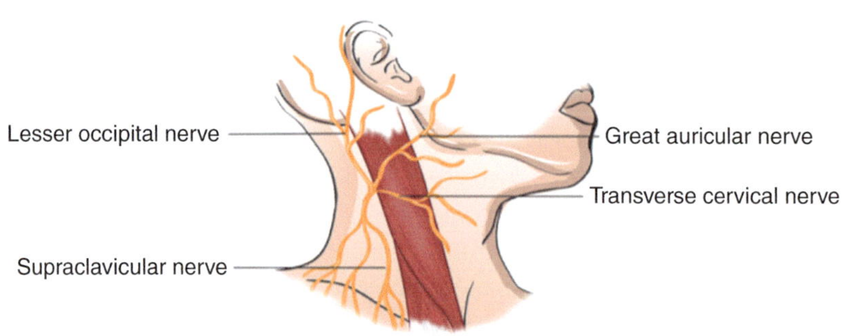

plexus anastomoses with the spinal accessory nerve, hypoglossal nerve, facial nerve, vagus nerve, glossopharyngeal nerve, and sympathetic trunk [16–20].

## Ultrasound Anatomy

The CP can be visualized as small hypoechoic oval structures deep or lateral to the posterior border of the SCM; however, this is not always visible [11] (Figs. 4, 5, 6, and 7). The important thing is that the phrenic nerve also is located in that area. The greater auricular nerve can usually be seen over the SCM [4].

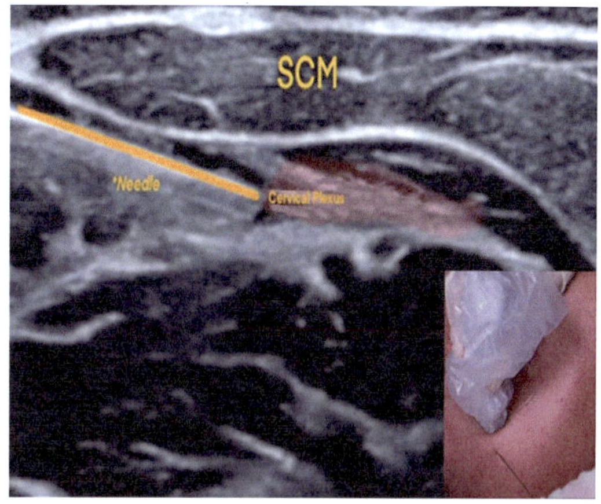


**Fig. 5** Probe position and an ultrasound image of the cervical plexus block. SCM sternocleidomastoid muscle.

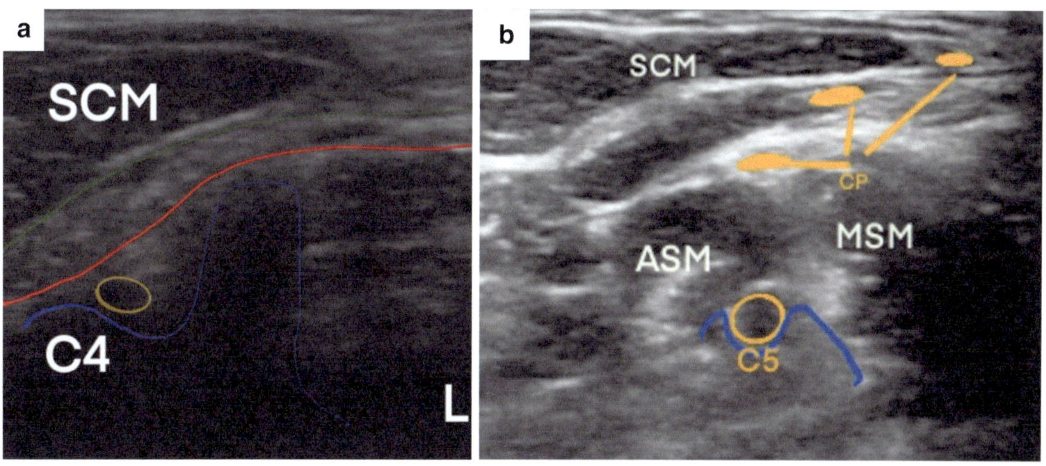


**Fig. 4** Ultrasound image of the cervical plexus. (**a**) SCM sternocleidomastoid muscle. Green line: investing layer of deep cervical fascia. Red line: prevertebral fascia L: lateral (**b**) SCM sternocleidomastoid muscle, ASM anterior scalene muscle, MSM middle scalene muscle, CP cervical plexus

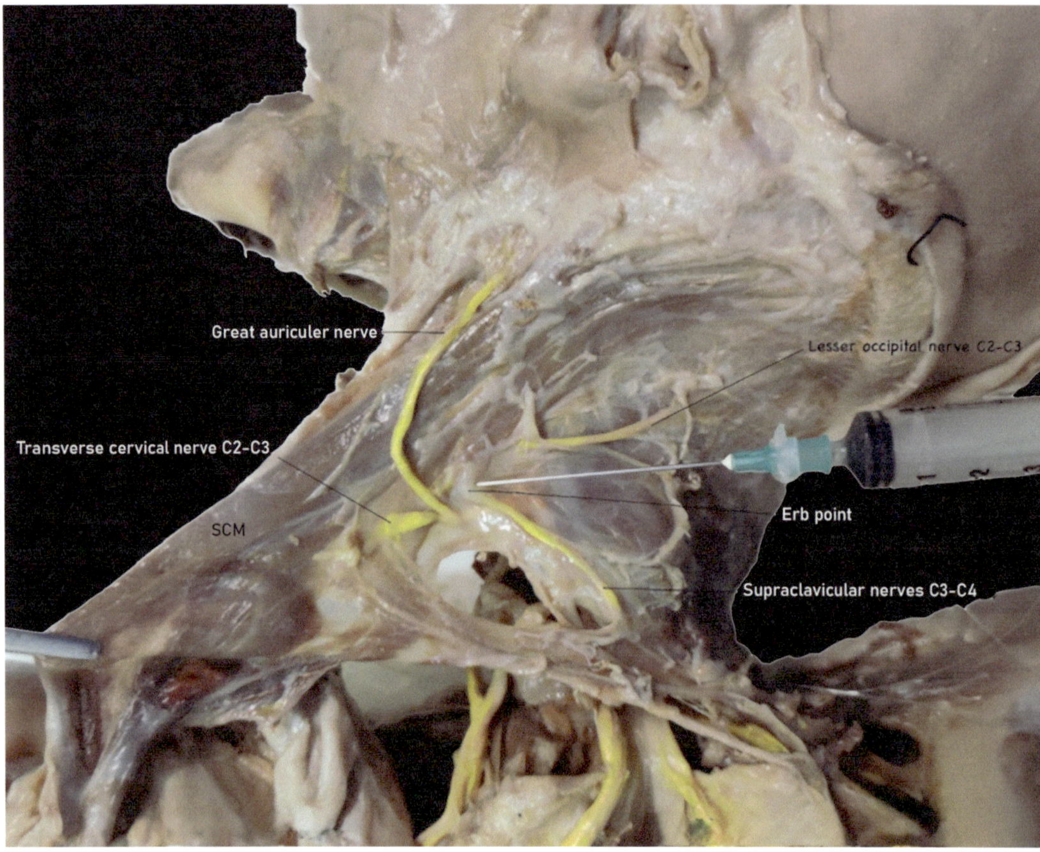


**Fig. 6** Superficial cutaneous branches of the cervical plexus on a cadaveric model

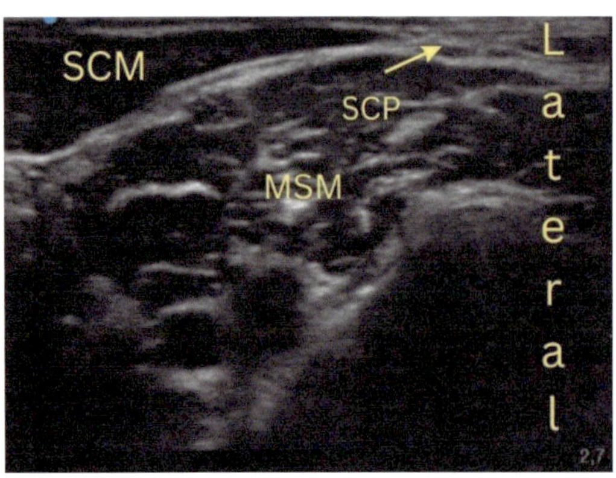


**Fig. 7** Ultrasound image of superficial cutaneous branches of cervical plexus. SCM sternocleidomastoid muscle, SCP superficial cutaneous branches of cervical plexus, MSM middle scalene muscle

## Scanning Techniques and Equipment

The patient takes a supine, semi-sitting position with the head slightly contralateral to the side. Also, the lateral decubitus position can be used. The patient's comfort and limitations should be considered during which position is used. In obese patients, the visualization of the posterior border of the SCM can be difficult; therefore, it can be asked the patient lift his/her head off the bed to facilitate palpation of the posterior border of the SCM. The transducer is placed inside a sterile sheath, and the gel is applied generously between the transducer and the inside of the sheath. The transducer is wrapped in a rubber band to prevent transducer movement inside the sheath. The skin is prepped and draped. The sterile gel is applied on the skin's surface to avoid any air between the transducer and the skin. Routinely, sterile towels, sterile gloves, sterile gauze pads, and chlorhexidine for skin preparation are used during the performance of the block. Ten ml of local anesthetic (short-acting like lidocaine for skin anesthesia and longer-acting agents like bupivacaine or ropivacaine) is enough dose for the block. A 5 cm 23–25 gauge needle can be used while performing the block. The high-frequency linear probe (13–18 MHz transducer) in a transverse orientation for an in-plane approach is placed over the midpoint of the posterior border of the sternocleidomastoid (Fig. 5). Usually, the appropriate depth of the area is 3–4 cm, and the focus range is 2–3 cm on the ultrasound screen. Once the SCM has been identified, the transducer is advanced posteriorly at approximately the levels of C4. The cervical plexus appears at the posterior to the SCM and superficial to the prevertebral fascia overlying the interscalene groove (Figs. 4 and 5).

## Approaches to Cervical Plexus Blocks

### Superficial Cervical Plexus Block

The superficial cervical plexus block is known as a low-risk block because it is a subcutaneous injection technique. It is performed at the posterior border of the SCM. However, it can be performed with ultrasound guidance as well (Figs. 5 and 6). Additionally, the ultrasound-guided superficial block is not easy because visualizing superficial CP is not always evident. While applying the block, the needle tip position should be located in the subcutaneous tissue to avoid the adverse effect of the deep block. Although the landmark-based block is easy to perform, ultrasound guidance prevents deep needle insertion and inadvertent injection into surrounding structures in the neck, and it helps to visualize the spread of the local anesthetic. Scanning starts at the C7 level because identifying the C7 level is easier (no anterior tubercle); then the transducer is moved cranially, and the posterior border of the SCM is identified. Local anesthetic is injected superficially into the investing layer of the deep cervical fascia. This block is a field block and is often applied using a large volume of local anesthetic [19, 20].

### Intermediate Cervical Plexus Block

Kefalianakis et al. reported the first case of ultrasound-guided intermediate cervical plexus block targeting the area between SCM and anterior scalene muscle in 2005, also named as an anterior approach (Fig. 4b) [21, 22]. Choquet et al. reported that the intermediate cervical plexus block should target posterior cervical space at the C4 level [12]. For the posterior approach, the posterior cervical space has been described as the area between SCM and prevertebral fascia (Fig. 4a). The posterior space runs into sub-investing fascial space described by Pandit et al. [11] The most common technique is the posterior approach. Local anesthetic is injected at the C4–C5 level, between the prevertebral fascia and the investing layer of the deep cervical fascia, under the SCM. Although the intermediate CP block is a deeper block compared to the superficial CP block, both of them target the same superficial branches of the cervical plexus. Intermediate CP block provides anesthetic and analgesic effects because the cervical branches of the nerve supply the SCM, after piercing the prevertebral fascia, are anastomosed with the spinal accessory nerve at the posterior surface or inside the SCM muscle. Although the spinal accessory nerve has a sensory function, it is presumed that the cervical plexus (ansacervicalis) provides alternative motor innervation for the SCM along with the spinal accessory nerve. It is possible for the intermediate CP block to simultaneously block the four cutaneous branches of the cervical plexus and the sensory/motor branches of the cervical plexus that supply the SCM. Therefore, it provides adequate anesthesia and analgesia for neck surgeries involving manipulation. In this respect, it should be kept in mind that there may be some adverse effects when applying the intermediate CP block [21–26].

## Deep Cervical Plexus Block

The deep cervical plexus block is a complex regional block technique and targets the C2–C4 spinal nerves. This technique blocks superficial and deep branches of the cervical plexus [27–33]. For this block, there are different approaches. At first approach, the target field is just behind the carotid sheath at the carotid bifurcation [32]. The injection is not deeper as much as the classical deep cervical block. Therefore, it is relatively safe. The second approach targets interscalene groove based on Winnie's description at the C4 level (Fig. 4b) [33]. It has advantages for shoulder surgery. The third approach is the classical description; in this technique, the C4 level is the target level, and the transducer is moved posteriorly till the transverse process of C4 is identified (thumbs up sign) (Fig. 4a) [32]. Local anesthetic is injected under prevertebral fascia without specifically targeting the nerve roots (Fig. 8).

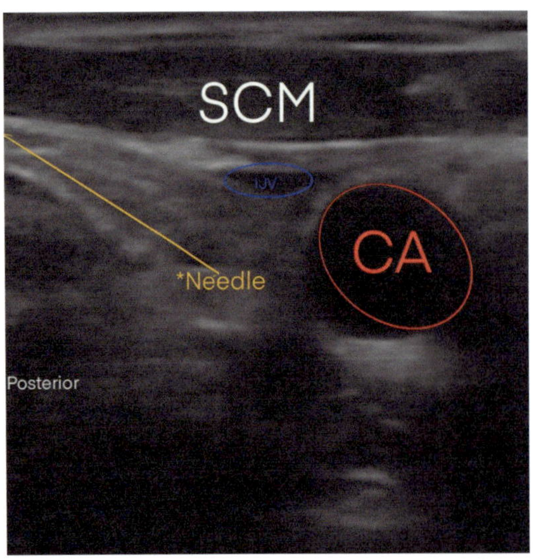


**Fig. 8** Carotid sheath field. CA Carotid artery, IJV Internal jugular vein, SCM sternocleidomastoid muscle

## Indication and Contraindications

The CP block can be performed for a variety of surgeries on the anterolateral neck to provide anesthesia and/or analgesia, parathyroidectomy, thyroidectomy, tympanomastoid surgery, anterior cervical fusion surgery, oral and maxillofacial surgery, and infratentorial and occipital craniotomy [34–41]. Additionally, the superficial cervical plexus block can be used as an adjuvant block for shoulder, breast, clavicle, lymph node dissections, upper chest wall surgeries, clavicular fractures, and central venous catheter placement [1, 42]. The carotid endarterectomy is the most common indication of the CP block [1]. The deep cervical plexus block can be used for neck pain and postoperative pain control after neck surgeries involving infrahyoid or SCM. Additionally, the deep CP block at the C2 or C3 level can be used for treating cervicogenic headaches [43]. Contraindications include patient refusal, morbid obesity, infection in the block area, contralateral phrenic nerve paralysis, radiotherapy on the neck, and allergies to local anesthetics. In patients with severe chronic obstructive pulmonary disease or untreated contralateral pneumothorax, caution should be exercised when performing this blog because it may inadvertently cause phrenic nerve dysfunction.

## Complications

Several complications can occur while performing the CP block. The superficial cervical block is relatively safe; therefore, the complications are related to any nerve block performed using local anesthetics, such as local anesthetic toxicity, intravascular injection, hematoma, and infection [44, 45]. The major complication of the CP block is phrenic nerve palsy [1]. However, this complication may not be seen all the time. Anatomic variations such as the dominance of the fifth cervical nerve and the presence/absence of the accessory phrenic nerve can be the reason why palsy is not seen in some patients. SCM is an accessory respiratory muscle and helps to breathe in diaphragmatic movement disorder, but since this muscle is relaxed by the deep cervical block, the diseases tend to worsen with this block, especially in patients with lung disease [1, 46–48]. With the advancement of technology, targeted areas and surrounding structures can be visualized better by ultrasound-guided techniques. As it is known, the intermediate cervical block is a deeper block compared to the superficial block and provides both anesthesia and analgesia. The literature explains why this partially deep block does not cause phrenic nerve palsy [1, 28, 49]. Seidel et al., in their study of fresh cadavers, suggested that since the intermediate cervical block is performed over prevertebral fascia at the posterior cervical space, prevertebral fascia could be protective against diaphragmatic palsy due to its impermeability feature to the local anesthetic [26, 50]. However, clinical studies are required to support this study.

The other complication is paralysis of the glossopharyngeal, hypoglossal, accessory nerves, and vagus [31, 50–67]. Although this complication is rare, this can occur during the deep CP block due to the spread of local anesthetic cephalad, and it causes fatal airway obstruction. Therefore, it is important to keep in mind that the deep CP block can lead not only to phrenic palsy but also to fatal airway obstruction. Consequently, preoperative routine history and examination of the patient with unilateral vocal cords or hypoglossal nerve palsy are important. It should be kept in mind that there may be complications such as temporary hoarseness, facial palsy, dysphagia, dyspnea, and Horner syndrome in the blocks made with the carotid sheath block approach or the blocks made with the anterior approach (in the interscalene groove) technique. During the intermediate CP block, the needle tip should be outside of the carotid sheath; thereby, the complication can be prevented.

## Clinical Pearls

Nomenclature cervical plexus block;

The superficial block is a safe, superficial, and easy-to-perform block. It is applied on the investing deep fascia. To see superficial branches can be difficult. Triangles of the neck, facial plan, bone structures, and SCM are the landmarks while applying an ultrasound-guided block.

The intermediate cervical block is applied between the investing deep fascia and the prevertebral fascia at the posterior cervical space. In order to prevent complications, it is important that the tip of the needle should not penetrate the prevertebral fascia and remain outside the carotid sheath.

The deep cervical block is performed under the prevertebral fascia by targeting the nerve roots. Care should be taken in terms of complications such as phrenic nerve palsy and fatal airway obstruction.

## References


1. Kim JS, Ko JS, Bang S, Kim H, Lee SY. Cervical plexus block. Korean J Anesthesiol. 2018a;71(4):274–88.
2. Winnie AP, Ramamurthy S, Durrani Z, Radonjic R. Interscalene cervical plexus block: a single-injection technic. Anesth Analg. 1975a;54:370–5.
3. Aunac S, Carlier M, Singelyn F, De Kock M. The analgesic efficacy of bilateral combined superficial and deep cervical plexus block administered before thyroid surgery under general anesthesia. Anesth Analg. 2002;95:746–50.
4. Christ S, Kaviani R, Rindfleisch F, Friederich P. Brief report: identification of the great auricular nerve by ultrasound imaging and transcutaneous nerve stimulation. Anesth Analg. 2012;114:1128–30.
5. Demondion X, Herbinet P, Boutry N, et al. Sonographic mapping of the normal brachial plexus. Am J Neuroradiol. 2003;24:1303–9
6. Eti Z, Irmak P, Gulluoglu BM, Manukyan MN, Gogus FY. Does bilateral superficial cervical plexus block decrease analgesic requirement after thyroid surgery? Anesth Analg. 2006;102:1174–6.
7. Flaherty J, Horn JL, Derby R. Regional anesthesia for vascular surgery. Anesthesiol Clin. 2014;32:639–59.
8. Guay J. Regional anesthesia for carotid surgery. Curr Opin Anaesthesiol. 2008;21:638–44.
9. Narouze S. Sonoanatomy of the cervical spinal nerve roots: implications for brachial plexus block. Reg Anesth Pain Med. 2009;34:616.
10. Telford RJ, Stoneham MD. Correct nomenclature of superficial cervical plexus blocks. Br J Anaesth. 2004;92:775.
11. Pandit JJ, Dutta D, Morris JF. Spread of injectate with superficial cervical plexus block in humans: an anatomical study. Br J Anaesth. 2003;91:733–5.
12. Choquet O, Dadure C, Capdevila X. Ultrasound-guided deep or intermediate cervical plexus block: the

target should be the posterior cervical space. Anesth Analg. 2010;111:1563–4.
13. Shakespeare TJ, Tsui BC. Intermittent hoarseness with continuous interscalene brachial plexus catheter infusion due to deficient carotid sheath. Acta Anaesthesiol Scand. 2013;57:1085–6.
14. Stecco A, Meneghini A, Stern R, Stecco C, Imamura M. Ultrasonography in myofascial neck pain: randomized clinical trial for diagnosis and follow-up. Surg Radiol Anat. 2014;36:243–53.
15. Tschopp KP, Gysin C. Local injection therapy in 107 patients with myofascial pain syndrome of the head and neck. ORL J Otorhinolaryngol Relat Spec. 1996;58:306–10.
16. Netter FH. Atlas of human anatomy. 6th ed. Philadelphia: Elsevier; 2014. PA: Churchill Livingstone: Elsevier
17. Morton D, Albertine K, Foreman B. The big picture: gross anatomy. New York: The McGraw-Hill Companies Inc.; 2011.
18. Roessel T, Wiessner D, Heller AR, et al. High-resolution ultrasound-guided high interscalene plexus block for carotid endarterectomy. Reg Anesth Pain Med. 2007;32:247–53.
19. Soeding P, Eizenberg N. Review article: anatomical considerations for ultrasound guidance for regional anesthesia of the neck and upper limb. Can J Anaesth. 2009;56:518–33.
20. Tran DQ, Dugani S, Finlayson RJ. A randomized comparison between ultrasound-guided and landmark-based superficial cervical plexus block. Reg Anesth Pain Med. 2010;35:539–43.
21. Kefalianakis F, Koeppel T, Geldner G, Gahlen J. Carotid-surgery in ultrasound-guided anesthesia of the regio colli lateralis. Anasthesiol Intensivmed Notfallmed Schmerzther. 2005;40:576–81.
22. Calderon AL, Zetlaoui P, Benatir F, Davidson J, Desebbe O, Rahali N, et al. Ultrasound-guided intermediate cervical plexus block for carotid endarterectomy using a new anterior approach: a two-centre prospective observational study. Anaesthesia. 2015;70:445–51.
23. Kim JS, Lee J, Soh EY, Ahn H, Oh SE, Lee JD, et al. Analgesic effects of ultrasound-guided serratus-intercostal plane block and ultrasound guided intermediate cervical plexus block after single-incision transaxillary robotic thyroidectomy: a prospective, randomized, controlled trial. Reg Anesth Pain Med. 2016;41:584–8.
24. Kim JS, Joe HB, Park MC, Ahn H, Lee SY, Chae YJ. Postoperative analgesic effect of ultrasound-guided intermediate cervical plexus block on unipolar sternocleidomastoid release with myectomy in pediatric patients with congenital muscular torticollis: a prospective, randomized controlled trial. Reg Anesth Pain Med. 2018b;43:634–40.
25. Leblanc I, Chterev V, Rekik M, Boura B, Costanzo A, Bourel P, et al. Safety and efficiency of ultrasound-guided intermediate cervical plexus block for carotid surgery. Anaesth Crit Care Pain Med. 2016;35:109–14.
26. Seidel R, Schulze M, Zukowski K, Wree A. Ultrasound-guided intermediate cervical plexus block. Anat Study Anaesth. 2015;64:446–50.
27. Usui Y, Kobayashi T, Kakinuma H, Watanabe K, Kitajima T, Matsuno K. An anatomical basis for blocking of the deep cervical plexus and cervical sympathetic tract using an ultrasound-guided technique. Anesth Analg. 2010;110:964–8.
28. Dhonneur G, Saidi NE, Merle JC, Asfazadourian H, Ndoko SK, Bloc S. Demonstration of the spread of injectate with deep cervical plexus block: a case series. Reg Anesth Pain Med. 2007;32:116–9.
29. Saranteas T, Kostopanagiotou GG, Anagnostopoulou S, Mourouzis K, Sidiropoulou T. A simple method for blocking the deep cervical nerve plexus using an ultrasound-guided technique. Anaesth Intensive Care. 2011;39:971–2.
30. Perisanidis C, Saranteas T, Kostopanagiotou G. Ultrasound-guided combined intermediate and deep cervical plexus nerve block for regional anaesthesia in oral and maxillofacial surgery. Dentomaxillofac Radiol. 2013;42:29945724.
31. Sandeman DJ, Griffiths MJ, Lennox AF. Ultrasound guided deep cervical plexus block. Anaesth Intensive Care. 2006;34:240–4.
32. Kumar SS. The cervical plexus: anatomy and ultrasound guided blocks. Anaesth Pain Intensive Care. 2015;19(3):323–32.
33. Winnie AP, et al. Interscalene cervical plexus block: a single-injection technic. Anesth Analg. 1975b;54(3):370–5.
34. Mayhew D, Sahgal N, Khirwadkar R, Hunter JM, Banerjee A. Analgesic efficacy of bilateral superficial cervical plexus block for thyroid surgery: meta-analysis and systematic review. Br J Anaesth. 2018;120:241–51.
35. Kannan S, Surhonne NS, Chethan Kumar C, Kavitha B, Devika Rani R, Raghavendra Rao RS. Effects of bilateral superficial cervical plexus block on sevoflurane consumption during thyroid surgery under entropy-guided general anesthesia: a prospective randomized study. Korean J Anesthesiol. 2018;71:141–8.
36. Girard F, Quentin C, Charbonneau S, Ayoub C, Boudreault D, Chouinard P, et al. Superficial cervical plexus block for transitional analgesia in infratentorial and occipital craniotomy: a randomized trial. Can J Anaesth. 2010;57:1065–70.
37. Pintaric TS, Hocevar M, Jereb S, Casati A, Novak JV. A prospective, randomized comparison between combined (deep and superficial) and superficial cervical plexus block with levobupivacaine for minimally invasive parathyroidectomy. Anesth Analg. 2007;105:1160–3.
38. Davies MJ, Silbert BS, Scott DA, Cook RJ, Mooney PH, Blyth C. Superficial and deep cervical plexus block for carotid artery surgery: a prospective study of 1000 blocks. Reg Anesth. 1997;22:442–6.

39. Ivanec Z, Mazul-Sunkol B, Lovricević I, Sonicki Z, Gvozdenović A, Klican K, et al. Superficial versus combined (deep and superficial) cervical plexus block for carotid endarterectomy. Acta Clin Croat. 2008;47:81–6.
40. Pandit JJ, Bree S, Dillon P, Elcock D, McLaren ID, Crider B. A comparison of superficial versus combined (superficial and deep) cervical plexus block for carotid endarterectomy: a prospective, randomized study. Anesth Analg. 2000;91:781–6.
41. SaitKavaklı A, KavrutÖztürk N, UmutAyoğlu R, Sağdıç K, Çakmak G, İnanoğlu K, et al. Comparison of combined (deep and superficial) and intermediate cervical plexus block by use of ultrasound guidance for carotid endarterectomy. J Cardiothorac Vasc Anesth. 2016;30:317–22.
42. Herring A. The ultrasound guided superficial cervical plexus block for anesthesia and analgesia in emergency care settings. Am J Emerg Med. 2012;30:1263–7.
43. Goldberg ME, Schwartzman RJ, Domsky R, Sabia M, Torjman MC. Deep cervical plexus block for the treatment of cervicogenic headache. Pain Physician. 2008;11:849–54.
44. GALA Trial Collaboratorive Group. General anaesthesia versus local anaesthesia for carotid surgery. Lancet. 2008;372:2213–142.
45. Martusevicius R. Ultrasound guided locoregionalanaesthesia for carotid endarterectomy. Eur J Vasc Endovasc Surg. 2012;44:27–30.
46. Pandit JJ, Satya-Krishna R, Gration P. Superficial or deep cervical plexus block for carotid endarterectomy: a systematic review of complications. Br J Anaesth. 2007;99:159–69.
47. Shin HJ, Yu HN, Yoon SZ. Ultrasound-guided subcutaneous cervical plexus block for carotid endarterectomy in a patient with chronic obstructive pulmonary disease. J Anesth. 2014;28:304–5.
48. Caliot P, Cabanié P, Bousquet V, Midy D. A contribution to the study of the innervation of the sternocleidomastoid muscle. Anat Clin. 1984;6:21–8.
49. Castresana MR, Masters RD, Castresana EJ, Stefansson S, Shaker IJ, Newman WH. Incidence and clinical significance of hemidiaphragmatic paresis in patients undergoing carotid endarterectomy during cervical plexus block anesthesia. J Neurosurg Anesthesiol. 1994;6:21–3.
50. Koizumi M, Horiguchi M, Sekiya S, Isogai S, Nakano M. A case of the human sternocleidomastoid muscle additionally innervated by the hypoglossal nerve. Okajimas Folia Anat Jpn. 1993;69:361–7.
51. Caliot P, Bousquet V, Midy D, Cabanié P. A contribution to the study of the accessory nerve: surgical implications. Surg Radiol Anat. 1989;11:11–5.
52. Tubbs RS, Sorenson EP, Watanabe K, Loukas M, Hattab E, Cohen-Gadol AA. Histologic confirmation of neuronal cell bodies along the spinal accessory nerve. Br J Neurosurg. 2014;28:746–9.
53. Bremner-Smith AT, Unwin AJ, Williams WW. Sensory pathways in the spinal accessory nerve. J Bone Joint Surg Br. 1999;81:226–8.
54. Pu YM, Tang EY, Yang XD. Trapezius muscle innervation from the spinal accessory nerve and branches of the cervical plexus. Int J Oral Maxillofac Surg. 2008;37:567–72.
55. Carling A, Simmonds M. Complications from regional anaesthesia for carotid endarterectomy. Br J Anaesth. 2000;84:797–800.
56. Campbell EJ. The role of the scalene and sternomastoid muscles in breathing in normal subjects; an electromyographic study. J Anat. 1955;89:378–86.
57. Lisboa C, Paré PD, Pertuzé J, Contreras G, Moreno R, Guillemi S, et al. Inspiratory muscle function in unilateral diaphragmatic paralysis. Am Rev Respir Dis. 1986;134:488–92.
58. Bonnevie T, Gravier FE, Ducrocq A, Debeaumont D, Viacroze C, Cuvelier A, et al. Exercise testing in patients with diaphragm paresis. Respir Physiol Neurobiol. 2018;248:31–5.
59. Stoneham MD, Wakefield TW. Acute respiratory distress after deep cervical plexus block. J Cardiothorac Vasc Anesth. 1998;12:197–8.
60. Lookman AA. Brachial plexus infiltration; single injection technique. Anaesthesia. 1958;13:5–18.
61. Warshafsky D, Goldenberg D, Kanekar SG. Imaging anatomy of deep neck spaces. Otolaryngol Clin N Am. 2012;45:1203–21.
62. Shibata Y, Fujiwara Y, Komatsu T. A new approach of ultrasound-guided stellate ganglion block. Anesth Analg. 2007;105:550–1.
63. Urmey WF, Talts KH, Sharrock NE. One hundred percent incidence of hemidiaphragmatic paresis associated with interscalene brachial plexus anesthesia as diagnosed by ultrasonography. Anesth Analg. 1991;72:498–503.
64. Suzuki S, Yasunaga H, Matsui H, Fushimi K, Saito Y, Yamasoba T. Factors associated with neck hematoma after thyroidectomy: a retrospective analysis using a Japanese inpatient database. Medicine (Baltimore). 2016;95:e2812.
65. Carmichael FJ, McGuire GP, Wong DT, Crofts S, Sharma S, Montanera W. Computed tomographic analysis of airway dimensions after carotid endarterectomy. Anesth Analg. 1996;83:12–7.
66. Kwok OK, Sun KO, Ahchong AK, Chan CK. Airway obstruction following carotid endarterectomy. Anaesth Intensive Care. 2004;32:818–20.
67. Zhang M, Lee AS. The investing layer of the deep cervical fascia does not exist between the sternocleidomastoid and trapezius muscles. Otolaryngol Head Neck Surg. 2002;127:452–4.

# Cervical Facet and Medial Branch Blocks

Kamal Mezian and Ondřej Naňka

## Background

Pain originating from the cervical zygapophyseal joint (also known as the facet joint) plays an important role in the diagnosis of chronic pain in the head, neck, shoulder, periscapular, and supraclavicular regions. Facetogenic pain is generally poorly defined. Its radiation does not follow a dermatomal distribution, and there is no motor or sensory deficit (unless there is a coexisting condition coupled with the symptoms mentioned above). The prevalence of facetogenic pain in patients with chronic neck pain was reported to be 36–55% [1, 2]. As the most common symptomatic, the C2–C3 and C5–C6 facet joints were identified [3]. Facet joint osteoarthritis (OA) is a common abnormality on plain radiographs of patients older than 60 years [4]. Notably, the association between OA of the zygapophyseal joint and pain is controversial and, to this date, remains a matter of debate. Another possible cause of facetogenic pain is strain during a whiplash injury [5]. Patients resistant to noninvasive conservative approaches (exercise therapy, physical agents, soft tissue/spinal manipulation techniques, pharmacotherapy, ergonomy/activity modification, and behavioral/psychotherapy) may benefit from a targeted injection, possibly improving functioning and providing pain relief [6]. The widely accepted gold standard to verify facetogenic pain as the primary source of nociception is a diagnostic image-guided anesthetic block targeting medial branch nerve fibers [7]. Variations in its course underline the importance of ultrasound (US) guidance when targeting the medial branch [8]. Therapeutic interventional procedures could target the anticipated pain generators: intra- and periarticular components of the facet joints or/and the medial branch nerve fibers. These procedures are third occipital nerve and medial branch radiofrequency neurotomy, cryoablation and injections (potentially also using neurolytic agents), and intraarticular facet joint injections. Notably, a multidisciplinary (rehabilitation) team approach is necessary to achieve the optimal treatment outcome.

K. Mezian (✉)
Department of Rehabilitation Medicine, First Faculty of Medicine, Charles University and General University Hospital, Prague, Czech Republic

O. Naňka
Institute of Anatomy, First Faculty of Medicine, Charles University, Prague, Czech Republic
e-mail: Ondrej.Nanka@lf1.cuni.cz

## Anatomy

The paired synovial facet joints are located on either side of the posterior aspect of the vertebral column (Fig. 1). These joints are formed by opposing inferior and superior articular processes that arise from the pedicle lamina junc-



T. Akkaya, A. Cömert (eds.), *Practical Guide for Pain Interventions: Head and Neck Sonoanatomy*,
https://doi.org/10.1007/978-3-031-88773-4_12

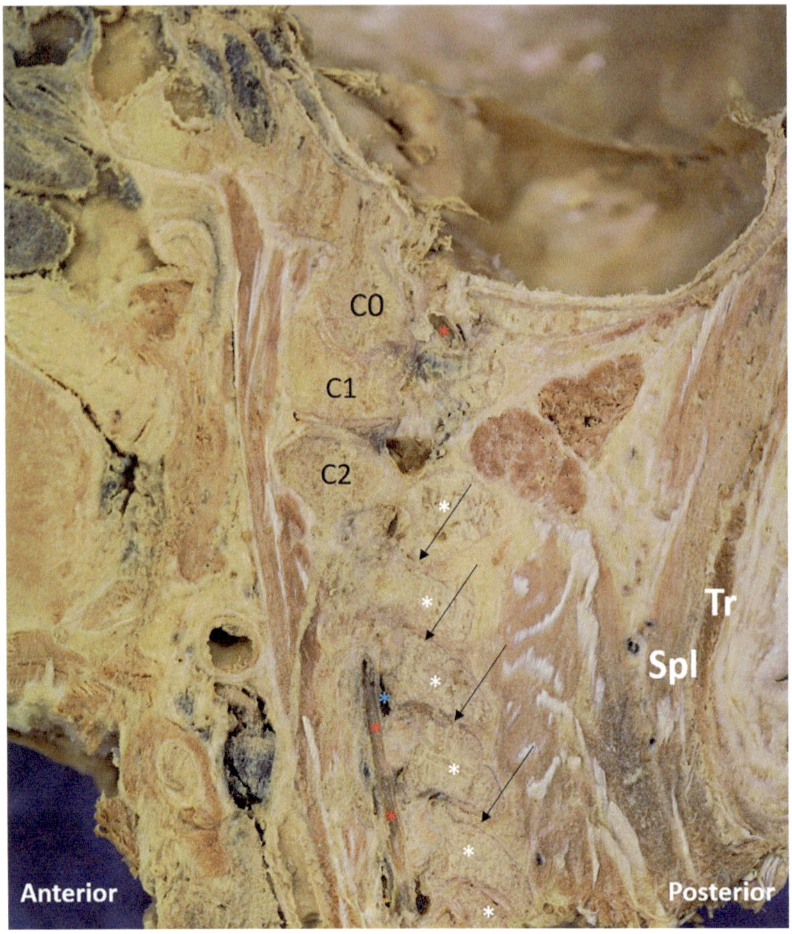


**Fig. 1** The parasagittal section on the cadaveric specimen demonstrates facet joint topography. The joint space *(black arrows)* of the cervical facet joints varies in its angle of inclination, depending on the level. C: cervical vertebral body, white asterisk: articular process, tr: trapezius, spl: splenius, red asterisk: vertebral artery, blue asterisk: vertebral vein

tion of two adjacent vertebrae. They are synovial diarthrodial joints with a thin hyaline cartilage layer covering both opposing articular surfaces [9]. The true joint capsule consists of the synovial and fibrous layers. Notably, anteriorly, the joint capsule represents the posterior boundary for the intervertebral foramina, defining this important mutual relationship. Furthermore, a 'meniscus-like' structure and subcapsular fat are commonly present intra-articularly [10, 11]. The size, shape, and joint gap inclination depend on the level. The narrow joint space is angulated approximately 45 degrees to the horizontal plane in the upper cervical spine. At the same time, the angle becomes more vertical in the lower part of the cervical spine, progressively from C3 to T1. Notably, right-to-left asymmetry is common concerning the articulation angle [9]. Regarding orientation in the transverse plane, the C2–C3 facets are oriented posteromedially, while when moving caudally, a gradual change to posterolateral is observed. Facet joints allow for subtle mobility between vertebrae [12]. The capsule of the facet joints, the synovium, its fold, and subchondral bone are extensively innervated; and represent an important source of pain sensation and proprioception [13]. Notably, each facet joint receives a dual innervation supply from the dorsal rami of two different spinal levels, at the corresponding level and from the above segment [14]. These articular fibers originate from the medial branches of the dorsal rami (Fig. 2). These C3–C7 dorsal rami run dorsally from the transverse process of the corresponding vertebra. The medial branches of each cervical vertebral level wrap around the corresponding

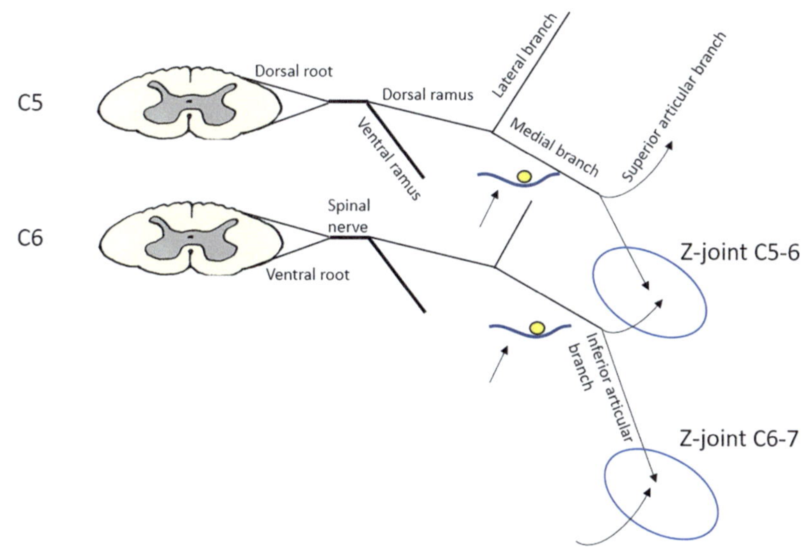


**Fig. 2** A schematic diagram demonstrating innervation of the cervical facet joint by medial branches of the dorsal rami of cervical nerves. The medial branch can be visualized with ultrasound at the waist of the articular pillar *(black arrow)*. Z-joint: zygapophysial joint

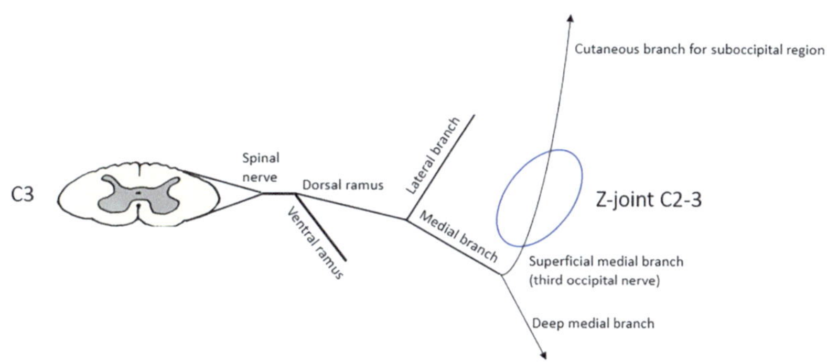


**Fig. 3** A schematic diagram shows the innervation of the C2–C3 facet joint by the third occipital nerve. Z-joint: zygapophysial joint

articular pillar [15]. For completeness, it should be noted that the C2–C3 facet joint receives innervation mainly from the superficial medial branch of the C3 dorsal ramus, also known as the third occipital nerve (Fig. 3), which should be targeted in selected cases (particularly when an association with headache is considered) [16]. This nerve runs dorsomedially adjacent to the superior articular process of the C3 vertebra and superficially becomes a cutaneous nerve, providing innervation of the suboccipital skin.

## Scanning Technique

The patient is placed in the lateral decubitus position with a small pillow below the ear. The prone position is also possible, mainly to visualize the facet joint capsule/joint gap. A pillow beneath the chest allows for slight flexion of the cervical spine when using the prone position. A high-frequency linear transducer is usually preferred. A curvilinear transducer can also be used depending on the patient's neck size. Several osseous structures provide important landmarks for orientation. The gain should be adjusted to clearly differentiate the bony surface. When the probe is placed at the midline in the longitudinal plane concerning the spine, with the superior end of the transducer on the occiput, the bifid spinous process of the C2 vertebra can be identified. When the probe is moved laterally, the vertebral lamina is observed. Laterally, facet joints are seen as 'sawtooth' or 'hill'-like structures, and articular pillars appear as depressions between them, sometimes called 'grooves' or 'valleys' [17]. Using Doppler imaging, the vertebral artery can be visualized between the transverse processes of

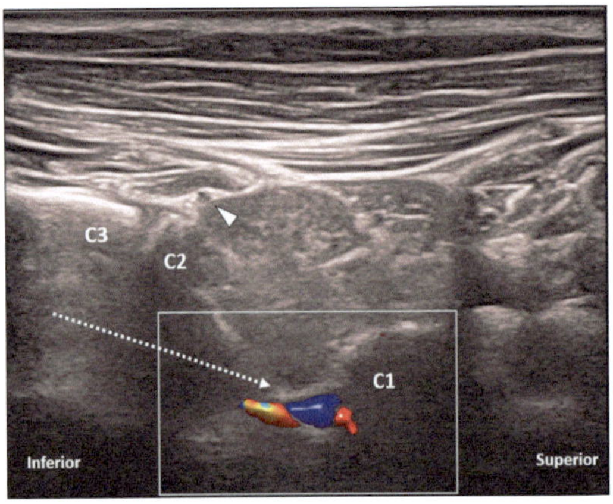


**Fig. 4** A sonographic image of the upper cervical spine shows the facet joint C2–C3. A hypoechoic third occipital nerve *(white arrowhead)* can be observed at the top of the C2 inferior articular pillar. Using Doppler imaging, the vertebral artery *(white dotted line)* can be identified pulsating between the C1 and C2 vertebrae

C1 and C2 (Fig. 4). Counting the facets starting from the articular pillar of C2 (axis), the proper level can be easily determined. Of note, sono palpation of the facet joints at individual levels can be used to assess for tenderness [18]. Scanning can also begin from the temporal bone mastoid process in the long axis. Moving the transducer in a posterior direction, the arch of C1 and the articular pillar of C2 can be seen. When the transducer is moved in the inferior direction, the joints of the upper cervical facet are identified. The superior and inferior articular processes that form the facet joints are seen as two hyperechoic bony echoes that give acoustic shadowing. The anechoic gap between them represents the joint space—the 'joint gap view' (Fig. 5). It should be noted that scanning can also reveal fluid and synovial thickening in the facet joint [18]. Rotating the ultrasound transducer in the direction of the external auditory meatus, the medial branch can be observed in its short axis as a hypoechoic ovoid structure at the deep points of the 'valleys' (articular pillars) between adjacent 'hills' (facet joints) and 'the medial branch view' (Fig. 6). The C7 medial branch is located more deeply and closer to the foramen. Thus, the nerve can be visualized between the transverse process and the articular pillar [19]. However, due to its deeper location, US visibility is suboptimal [20]. Another exception would be the third occipital nerve, which is visualized more laterally as a hypoechoic bubble above the top of the inferior articular process C2 [21].

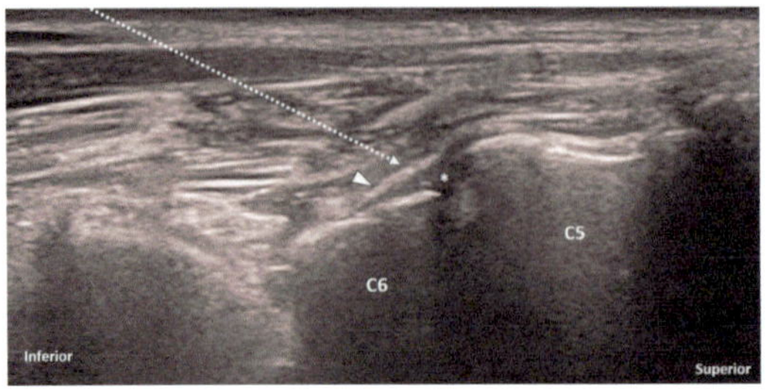


**Fig. 5** Short-axis ultrasound image of the medial branch—medial branch view. The medial branch *(white arrowhead)* shows a hypoechoic appearance at the deepest point of the 'valley' between the clefts, representing entry into the joint space *(white asterisks)*. The needle tip is placed perineurally *(white dotted line)*

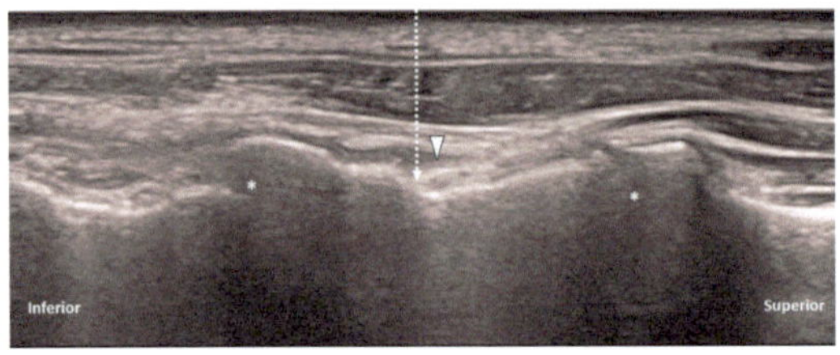


**Fig. 6** Ultrasound image of facet joint space—joint gap view. The C5–C6 facet joint space *(white asterisks)* is seen as a hypoechoic cleft between the C5 and C6 articular pillars. A joint capsule *(white arrowhead)* that covers the joint gap needs to be pierced during intraarticular injection *(white dotted line)*

## Ultrasound-Guided Procedures for Facetogenic Pain

### Injection of the Medial Branch and Third Occipital Nerve

The medial branch and the third occipital nerve can be targeted for diagnostic and therapeutic purposes. The US-guided technique is an analog for radiofrequency neurotomy and injection of drug solutions. When targeting the medial branch, it should be injected at two individual levels—at the spinal level of the affected facet joint and the above segment. For the third occipital nerve injection, the technique is similar to that of the medial branch, but the target is adjacent to the C2–3 facet joint. Furthermore, for the C2–3 facet joint block, a single injection is usually sufficient to influence most of its innervation. For the intervention, the patient is placed in the lateral decubitus position with the symptomatic side up. Using the 'medial branch view,' as described in the previous section, the proper medial branch is identified and visualized in the short axis and injected using the out-of-plane technique. Alternatively, the in-plane approach can be used based on personal preference [22]. After the pre-procedure scan and skin prep, the needle is inserted from anterior to posterior, adjacent to the hypoechoic dot, which represents the medial branch. It should be noted that the anterior-to-posterior direction of the needle is advantageous in preventing unintentional puncture of the anterior neck vasculature [16]. First, an aspiration should be performed to avoid intravascular injection. Afterward, 0.5 ml of the drug solution is administered perineurally. Depending on the purpose of the injection, a local anesthetic or a mixture with corticosteroids (or other drugs) can be used.

## Intraarticular Facet Joint Injection

The technique for intraarticular facet joint injection is feasible, but data on its clinical efficacy are insufficient [23, 24]. The patient is placed in the prone position with a pillow under his chest to allow a slight flexion of the neck to facilitate the US scan. Using the joint gap view described above, the proper facet joint is identified and visualized. Depending on personal preference, an in-plane or out-of-plane approach can be used. The direction of the needle trajectory can be superior to inferior or inferior to superior concerning the angle of inclination of the articular surface. After the pre-procedure scan and skin prep, the needle is advanced toward the hypoechoic cleft, representing the entry into the joint cavity. After piercing the joint capsule and preventive aspiration, 0.25 ml of the drug solution is slowly administered to the joint space. Depending on the suspected etiology, local anesthetics or/and corticosteroids can be used.

## Complications

A sudden and transient increase in pain is not uncommon after the procedures described above. Vascular puncture and intravascular injection are possible due to proximity to the vertebral artery, which runs anteriorly to the facet joint. Other severe adverse reactions are the result of unintentional spinal canal entry. In particular, the administration of local anesthetics to the foramen magnum could result in total spinal anesthesia with quadriplegia and respiratory failure [15, 25]. Trauma to the cervical nerve roots, which are located anterior to the facet joints, is also possible. After the procedure, patients should be observed for at least 30 minutes.

**Author Disclosures** Conflict of interest: Supported by MH CZ DRO-VFN 64165.

The anatomical specimen picture was elaborated using a donated body with the approval of the Institute of Anatomy of the First Faculty of Medicine, Charles University, Prague. Informed consent had been obtained from the donor.

## References

1. Speldewinde GC, Bashford GM, Davidson IR. Diagnostic cervical zygapophyseal joint blocks for chronic cervical pain. Med J Aust. 2001;174:174–6.
2. Manchikanti L, Boswell MV, Singh V, Pampati V, Damron KS, Beyer CD. Prevalence of facet joint pain in chronic spinal pain of cervical, thoracic, and lumbar regions. BMC Musculoskelet Disord. 2004;5:15.
3. Cooper G, Bailey B, Bogduk N. Cervical zygapophysial joint pain maps. Pain Med. 2007;8:344–53.
4. Eubanks JD, Lee MJ, Cassinelli E, Ahn NU. Prevalence of lumbar facet arthrosis and its relationship to age, sex, and race: an anatomic study of cadaveric specimens. Spine (Phila Pa 1976). 2007;32:2058–62.
5. Winkelstein BA, Nightingale RW, Richardson WJ, Myers BS. The cervical facet capsule and its role in whiplash injury: a biomechanical investigation. Spine (Phila Pa 1976). 2000;25:1238–46.
6. Manchikanti L, Hirsch JA, Kaye AD, Boswell MV. Cervical zygapophysial (facet) joint pain: effectiveness of interventional management strategies. Postgrad Med. 2016;128:54–68.

7. Barnsley L, Bogduk N. Medial branch blocks are specific for the diagnosis of cervical zygapophyseal joint pain. Reg Anesth. 1993;18:343–50.
8. Büsken F, Lataster A, Herrler A. The innervation of the cervical facet joints-an anatomical and histological approach. Clin Anat. 2022;35(6):780–8.
9. Cramer GD, Darby SA. Clinical anatomy of the spine, spinal cord, and ANS. St. Louis: Elsevier Health Sciences; 2017.
10. FFPM(ANZCA) NBBsMBMPDsDDFF. Clinical and radiological anatomy of the lumbar spine. 5th ed. Edinburgh; New York: Churchill Livingstone; 2012.
11. Farrell SF, Osmotherly PG, Cornwall J, Sterling M, Rivett DA. Cervical spine meniscoids: an update on their morphological characteristics and potential clinical significance. Eur Spine J. 2017;26:939–47.
12. DSc SSP, editor. Gray's anatomy: the anatomical basis of clinical practice. 42nd ed. Amsterdam: Elsevier; 2020.
13. Kallakuri S, Li Y, Chen C, Cavanaugh JM. Innervation of cervical ventral facet joint capsule: histological evidence. World J Orthop. 2012;3:10–4.
14. Bogduk N, Long DM. The anatomy of the so-called "articular nerves" and their relationship to facet denervation in the treatment of low-back pain. J Neurosurg. 1979;51:172–7.
15. Waldman SD. Atlas of interventional pain management. 5th ed. Philadelphia: Elsevier; 2020.
16. Narouze SN, editor. Atlas of ultrasound-guided procedures in interventional pain management. 2nd ed. New York: Springer; 2018.
17. Özçakar L. Ultrasound imaging & guidance for musculoskeletal interventions in physical and rehabilitation medicine. Milan: Edi Ermes; 2019.
18. Bodor M, Murthy N, Uribe Y. Ultrasound-guided cervical facet joint injections. Spine J. 2022;22:983–92. S1529-9430(22)00022-5
19. Chang K-V, Kara M, Su DC-J, Gürçay E, Kaymak B, Wu W-T, et al. Sonoanatomy of the spine: a comprehensive scanning protocol from cervical to sacral region. Med Ultrason. 2019;21:474–82.
20. Siegenthaler A, Schliessbach J, Curatolo M, Eichenberger U. Ultrasound anatomy of the nerves supplying the cervical zygapophyseal joints: an exploratory study. Reg Anesth Pain Med. 2011;36:606–10.
21. Li J, Szabova A. Ultrasound-guided nerve blocks in the head and neck for chronic pain management: the anatomy, sonoanatomy, and procedure. Pain Physician. 2021;24:533–48.
22. Finlayson RJ, Gupta G, Alhujairi M, Dugani S, Tran DQH. Cervical medial branch block: a novel technique using ultrasound guidance. Reg Anesth Pain Med. 2012;37:219–23.
23. Freire V, Grabs D, Lepage-Saucier M, Moser TP. Ultrasound-guided cervical facet joint injections: a viable substitution for fluoroscopy-guided injections? J Ultrasound Med. 2016;35:1253–8.
24. Falco FJE, Manchikanti L, Datta S, Wargo BW, Geffert S, Bryce DA, et al. Systematic review of the therapeutic effectiveness of cervical facet joint interventions: an update. Pain Physician. 2012;15:E839–68.
25. Lee H-I, Park Y-S, Cho T-G, Park S-W, Kwon J-T, Kim Y-B. Transient adverse neurologic effects of spinal pain blocks. J Korean Neurosurg Soc. 2012;52:228–33.

# Ultrasound-Guided Cervical Sympathetic Block

Semih Gungor and Burcu Candan

## Introduction

Ultrasound (US) use has gained popularity in interventional pain management practice in recent decades. Ultrasound-guided (USG) visualization of needles, nerves, blood vessels, and soft tissues can assist the interventionalist in real-time needle advancement. Thus, it may prevent inadvertent tissue trauma and intravascular and intraneural injections [13, 34, 36, 43], allow visualization of medication spread, and reduce the local anesthetic dose required to achieve reliable blockade [22, 23, 28]. Unlike fluoroscopy or CT-guided injections, there is no radiation risk for patients and medical staff during USG injections. The other advantages of USG are its availability for in-office use, portability, and relatively favorable cost compared to fluoroscopy or CT units. However, it must be emphasized that the safety and accuracy of USG interventions depend on the practitioners' training and experience.

**Table 1** The Advantages of Ultrasound Guided Cervical Sympathetic Block

| |
|---|
| Safer than blind and fluoroscopy guided technique |
| Reduces the required volume of local anesthetic |
| Minimize the risk of intravascular injection |
| Minimize the risk of vessel injury and hematoma formation |
| Minimize the risk of temporary paralysis of the recurrent laryngeal nerve: |
| Help to avoid applying improper injections |
| Minimize the risk of esophageal injury |
| Minimize the risk of mediastinitis |

Cervical sympathetic block (CSB) is a commonly used procedure for diagnostic or therapeutic purposes in various conditions, including neuropathic pain and sympathetically maintained pain, which may be a subgroup of complex regional pain syndrome (CRPS) involving the head, face, neck, and upper extremities [1].

The advantages are discussed in Table 1.

This chapter will review the indications, anatomy, sonoanatomy, techniques, advantages, disadvantages, and limitations of USG-CSB.

## Indications

CSB has been used for several indications for decades in pain management practice. These indications are:

S. Gungor
Division of Musculoskeletal and Interventional Pain Management, Department of Anesthesiology, Critical Care and Pain Management, Hospital for Special Surgery, New York, New York, USA

Department of Anesthesiology, Weill Cornell Medicine, New York, New York, USA

B. Candan (✉)
Division of Musculoskeletal and Interventional Pain Management, Department of Anesthesiology, Critical Care and Pain Management, Hospital for Special Surgery, New York, New York, USA



T. Akkaya, A. Cömert (eds.), *Practical Guide for Pain Interventions: Head and Neck Sonoanatomy*,
https://doi.org/10.1007/978-3-031-88773-4_13

- The diagnosis and treatment of sympathetically maintained pain and CRPS of the head, face, neck, and arms [25, 27, 47, 49].
- Central pain (e.g., post-stroke pain) [31, 46, 49]
- Postoperative pain [48]
- Pain after plexus injury [16]
- Neuropathic pain, including trigeminal or *postherpetic neuralgia* [10, 16, 27] *and phantom limb pain* [27]
- Diagnosis and management of peripheral vascular diseases, including *peripheral arterial disease* and *Raynaud's disease* [16]
- Cancer pain [8, 27]
- Orofacial pain [8, 20, 21, 40]
- Vascular headache, migraine [32]

CSB can also be used for different indications other than pain management, including the following conditions:

- Hyperhidrosis [16]
- Sudden sensory-neural hearing loss [16]
- Peripheral vascular disease [16]
- Ventricular dysrhythmias, including long-QT syndrome [16, 48]
- Panic and anxiety symptoms [33]
- Relief of hot flushes in postmenopausal patients and breast cancer survivors [29, 30]

## Contraindications

### Absolute Contraindications [1]

- Patient refusal
- Allergic reactions to local anesthetics
- Primary and secondary coagulopathy

### Relative Contraindications [1]

- A recent cardiac infarction and a severe cardiac conduction block: CSB may deteriorate cardiac function.
- Glaucoma: CSB may aggravate glaucoma.

## Anatomy

The preganglionic and postganglionic sympathetic nerves transmit sympathetic outflow from the spinal cord. The preganglionic fibers that arise from thoracic segments (T1–T4 spinal levels) progress to the cephalad and exit the ventral roots to join the cervical sympathetic chain by synapsing with superior, middle, and inferior cervical sympathetic ganglia and provide the sympathetic innervation of the head, neck, and upper extremities [9, 14]. The cervicothoracic (stellate) ganglion is formed by the fusion of the inferior cervical ganglion with the first thoracic ganglion [13, 24]. The stellate ganglion is located within the fascial plane of the prevertebral fascia, covered by the longus colli muscle, and is adjacent to the first rib at the level of T1 [17]. The CSB is typically performed at the C6 or C7 levels. The CSB primarily blocks the cervical sympathetic chain close to the middle cervical sympathetic ganglion at the C6 or C7 levels. Therefore, commonly used terminology like "stellate ganglion block" is a misnomer, as the block of stellate ganglion depends on the medication spreading from C6 or C7 levels to a more caudal location at the level of 1st rib. Thus, this chapter will use CSB instead of the well-known term "stellate ganglion block."

A local anesthetic block of the cervical sympathetic chain leads to a complete blockade of sympathetic supply to the ipsilateral head and neck but only partially to the ipsilateral upper limb. The anatomic variations reported in cadaveric studies indicated that the sympathetic nerves from the second thoracic (T2) and third thoracic (T3) ganglia could bypass the cervical sympathetic chain, including stellate ganglion, and directly connect to the brachial plexus in 20% of the population. In this population, CSB may fail to provide complete sympathetic blockade in the upper extremity [9, 14]. Knowledge about the anatomy of vascular structures of the area is vital for the safety of administering the CSB. The proximity of the vertebral artery, the thyrocervical trunk of the subclavian artery, the inferior thyroid artery, the carotid artery, and the jugular vein to the injection area is a significant safety concern during the CSB.

- The vertebral artery branches from the subclavian artery and ascends in the neck before entering the transverse foramen at C5 or C6. In most anatomical studies, the vertebral artery enters the transverse foramen at the level of C6. The remaining variations enter the transverse foramen at C5 and sometimes higher levels [15, 24]. The vertebral artery is in the needle pathway during CSB and is vulnerable to damage and intravascular injections, resulting in loss of consciousness, seizures, or stroke.
- The thyrocervical trunk of the subclavian artery ascends (running in front of the vertebral artery and the longus colli muscle) and follows a variable pathway.
- The inferior thyroid artery is also located at the base of the neck and may be in the needle pathway if an anterior approach is used for CSB.

## Sonoanatomy

The commonly used approach to the stellate ganglion is at C6 and C7 levels, and USG can help improve the safety of CSB [12]. The main advantage of the USG-CSB is to allow the clinician to visualize critical vascular structures to determine the optimum needle pathway in real-time during the injection. Color Doppler function of the US can be utilized to evaluate vascular structures more effectively before the planned injection. Besides, the US can also allow visualization of the thyroid gland, C6 anterior and posterior tubercles, longus colli muscle, longus capitis muscle, prevertebral fascia, and esophagus [43]. The possibility of high variation in the thickness of the longus colli muscle was reported in anatomic and imaging studies and suggested that this variation may lead to failure in CSB [2]. The sympathetic ganglion is located directly over the longus colli muscle and below the prevertebral fascia. Therefore, the prevertebral superficial fascia is an essential target for advancing the needle tip and plays a critical role in spreading injectate to sympathetic ganglion during USG-CSB [18] (Figs. 2, 3, and 4). The ideal location for the needle tip is superficial to the longus colli muscle and between the two laminae of the prevertebral superficial fascia [37].

The vertebral artery can be visualized below the C6 before entering the transverse foramen. Clinicians should be aware of the anatomical variations of the vertebral artery. In anatomical studies, in about 10% of the cases, the vertebral artery may enter the foramen transversum at C5 and sometimes higher levels. At the C6 level, the cervical sympathetic chain is anterior to the longus colli muscle and posterior to the prevertebral fascia [43]. The inferior thyroidal artery is anterior to the prevertebral fascia [43].

The esophagus is another important structure that we can visualize during the CSB. The esophagus shows a variable course and mostly deviates to the left of the trachea (50–70%). In one study, Bhatia et al. reported the position of the esophagus lateral to the airway in 50% and 74% of the subjects at C6 and C7, respectively [5]. The esophagus has an oval shape and can be separated from other structures in the neck by observing peristaltic movements when the patient is asked to swallow.

## Patient Position

- The patient is placed supine with the neck slightly extended.
- The head is turned slightly opposite side.

## Ultrasound-Probe Position

- The operator's non-dominant hand can support the probe while the dominant hand manipulates the needle.
- The suggested point for placing the probe is the paramedian location at the base of the neck just above the projection of the medial end of the clavicle.

## Probe

- A high-frequency (6–15 MHz) linear transducer can be used for a more commonly preferred lateral to medial approach to USG-CSB.
  - This transducer is smaller than many curvilinear probes and allows in-plane needle visualization
- A *micro-size* curvilinear transducer (2.5–7 MHz) may be used for less commonly preferred anterior (medial to lateral) USG-CSB.
  - This transducer is small enough to fit between the carotid artery and trachea, allowing in-plane needle visualization.

## Probe Placement

### Lateral (Lateral to Medial) Approach (Figs. 1 and 2)

- The linear transducer must be placed horizontally at the level of C6 (approximately at the cricoid cartilage level in most subjects).
- A preliminary scan should be performed to evaluate the anatomical structures, including the anterior tubercle of C6, longus colli muscle, vascular structures, and esophagus.
- The anterior tubercle of the C6 transverse process and the transverse process of C7 that is seen below the tubercle are important key landmarks for confirming the location by moving the transducer caudally and cranially.
- The structures, including the longus colli muscle and prevertebral fascia, are essential for needle target.
- The vascular structures, including the internal jugular vein and carotid artery, are essential to determine the needle pathway in the lateral approach.
- The needle is directed between the internal jugular vein and the anterior tubercle of C6. The needle tip is positioned posterior to the prevertebral fascia and anterior to the longus colli muscle.
- 25 gauge, 3.5-inch spinal needle

### Anterior (Medial to Lateral) Approach (Figs. 3 and 4)

- A *micro-size* curvilinear transducer must be placed horizontally at the level of C6 (approximately at the cricoid cartilage level in most subjects).
- A preliminary scan should be performed to evaluate the anatomical structures, including the anterior tubercle of C6, longus colli muscle, vascular structures, and esophagus.

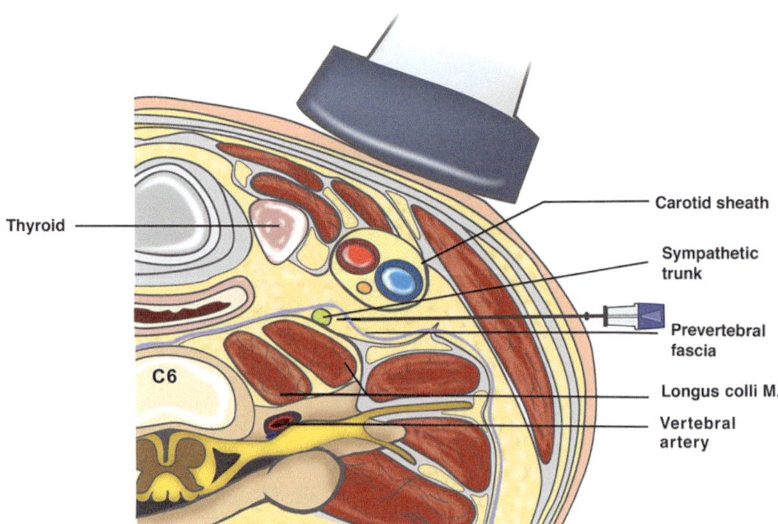


**Fig. 1** Illustration showing the position of the ultrasound probe and the needle in the lateral(lateral to medial) approach

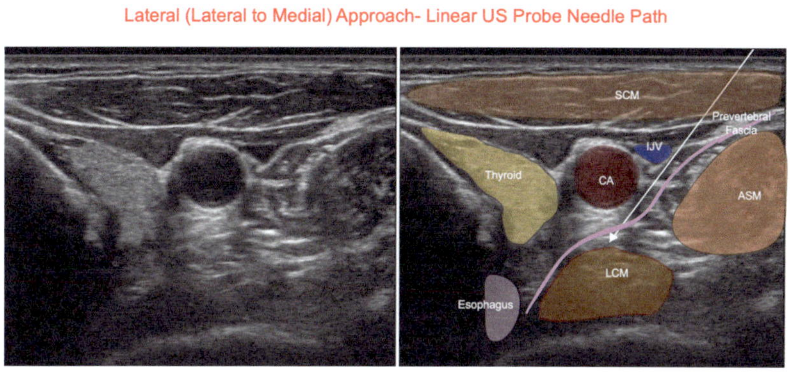


**Fig. 2** The USG image shows the needle pathway for lateral (lateral to medial) approach to the cervical sympathetic ganglion. The other medical structures in the image include the following: SCM Sternocleidomastoid Muscle, IJV Internal Jugular Vein, CA Carotid Artery, ASM Anterior Scalene Muscle, LCM Longus Colli Muscle

**Fig. 3** Illustration showing the position of the ultrasound probe and the needle in the anterior (medial to lateral) approach

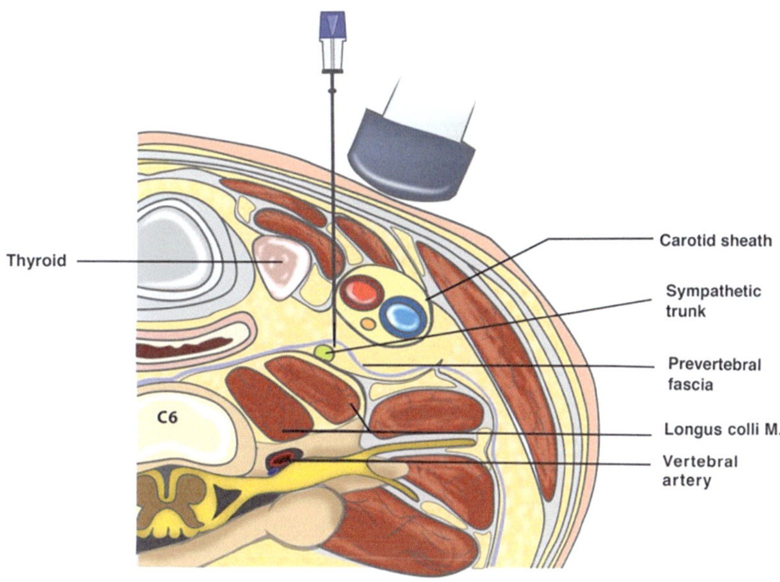


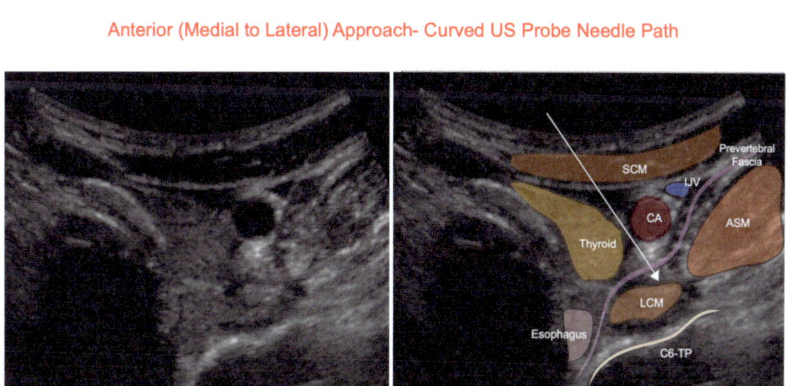


**Fig. 4** The USG image shows the needle pathway for anterior (medial to lateral) approach to the cervical sympathetic ganglion. The other medical structures in the US image include the following: SCM Sternocleidomastoid Muscle, IJV Internal Jugular Vein, CA Carotid Artery, ASM Anterior Scalene Muscle, LCM Longus Colli Muscle, TP Transverse Process

- The anterior tubercle of the C6 transverse process and the transverse process of C7 that is seen below the tubercle are important key landmarks for confirming the location by moving the transducer caudally and cranially.
- The structures, including the thyroid gland, carotid artery, longus colli muscle, and prevertebral fascia, are essential for needle target.
- The vascular structures, including the carotid artery, inferior thyroid artery, and vertebral artery, are important to determine the needle pathway in the anterior approach.
- The needle is directed between the carotid artery and trachea, and the needle tip is positioned posterior to the prevertebral fascia and anterior to the longus colli muscle.
- 25 gauge, 2.5-inch spinal needle.

## Procedure Approach

- The preliminary US scanning before the procedure is essential for determining the appropriate approach and orientation of the needle [5]. During the initial US scanning, all critical structures, including the carotid artery, internal jugular vein, thyroid gland, trachea, esophagus, longus colli muscle covered with the prevertebral fascia, C6 nerve, and transverse process of C6, must be identified (Figs. 2, 3, and 4). The C6 transverse process is identified by its prominent anterior tubercle (the anterior tubercle of C6 is known as Chassaignac's tubercle) [43].
- The common approaches are listed below [13, 37]:
  - Anterior (out-of-plane) with linear transducer,
  - Anterior, medial to lateral (in-plane with use of *micro-size* curvilinear transducer)
  - Lateral (in-plane) approaches.

The needle is directed between the trachea and the carotid artery for the anterior approach and passes through the thyroid gland. The anterior out-of-plane approach using a linear transducer is less popular in clinical practice due to the risk of vascular injury to the inferior thyroid and vertebral arteries [12, 27]. Besides, the needle tip may not be adequately visualized during the out-of-plane technique. An in-plane anterior approach using a *micro-size* curvilinear transducer allows better visualization of the needle tip than the out-of-plane anterior approach technique.

The commonly preferred approach is the lateral (in-plane) because it avoids the vascular structures during the needle placement. The lateral approach can be planned from the sternocleidomastoid muscle; the needle is directed from lateral to medial and passes lateral to the carotid artery and internal jugular vein [12, 26, 27].

- In a study, Gofeld et al. reported that the cervical sympathetic trunk lies entirely subfascial (posterior to the prevertebral fascia) at the C6 level; therefore, subfascial injection provides a reliable spread of a solution caudally to the stellate ganglion with less risk of complications [12, 13, 41]. Ultrasound guidance can help the clinician apply proper subfascial injection using real-time needle advancement. For subfascial injection, the needle tip is positioned between the prevertebral fascia and the longus colli muscle. In contrast, the spread of injectate to the suprafascial area tends to achieve cephalad, medial, and anterior spread. This approach can result in the blockade of recurrent laryngeal nerves, thereby the risk of hoarseness. Injections with subfascial orientation caused less hoarseness than injections with suprafascial orientation [41].

## Potential Risks of the Stellate Ganglion Blockade

The anatomical proximity of the carotid artery, inferior thyroid artery, trachea, and esophagus can be in the needle trajectory during CSB. Therefore, ultrasound guidance for CSB offers the additional advantage of real-time visualization of critical structures, including vessels (the inferior thyroid, vertebral, cervical, and carotid arteries), nerves, the esophagus, and the thyroid gland for safer injection. Moreover, the distribution of the injectate between the carotid sheath, thyroid, and esophagus can be monitored, and the needle position can be corrected when necessary.

The potential complications during the performance of USG-CSB can be listed as follows [39]:

### Intravascular Injection

There are critical vascular structures along the needle's pathway during CSB. These vascular structures are the vertebral artery, the thyrocervical trunk of the subclavian artery, the inferior thyroid artery, the carotid artery, and the internal jugular vein. Therefore, there is a risk of vessel puncture or intravascular injection during the CSB. Real-time ultrasound monitoring may potentially recognize these vascular structures to prevent blood vessel damage before it happens and recognize the inadvertent injection. The fluoroscopy-guidance technique can also help avoid unintentional drug injection only after the contrast is injected but does not help prevent blood vessel rupture. Inadvertent local anesthetic injection into a vertebral artery is an important risk as it can precipitate seizure activity, sudden loss of consciousness, or stroke [5]. The possibility of injection of local anesthetics to the vertebral artery is more likely at the C7 level because the vertebral artery is extraforaminal at this level and is exposed to the risk of puncture and local anesthetic injection. This is one of the main reasons why an injection at the C6 level is preferred during CSB.

The symptoms and signs associated with the intravascular injection can be listed as perioral tingling/numbness, tinnitus, dysarthria, convulsions, dysrhythmias, mental status changes, cardiovascular instability, and cardiopulmonary arrest [38]. The spread of local anesthetic into epidural space may cause hypotension, bradycardia, or total spinal block [1]. Another concern is particulate steroids mixed with local anesthetics during CSB, which can cause occlusive ischemia in end organs. Intraarterial injection of particulate steroids into the carotid or vertebral arteries may result in stroke, or injection into the cervical spinal segmental artery can result in spinal cord infarction [39].

### Vessel Injury and Hematoma Formation

Hematoma related to blood vessel injury is another potential complication of CSB. Retropharyngeal hematoma (RPH) is rare but can be a catastrophic complication of CSB. It can cause life-threatening airway obstruction [15, 44, 45]. Clinicians should be aware of the RPH symptoms, including pain in the neck, throat, chest, upper back, and upper airway symptoms. The procedure should be planned in suitable conditions for emergency airway management. Inferior thyroid artery injury is a significant cause of retropharyngeal hematoma [35]. The risk of injury to the inferior thyroid artery may be due to anatomical variations of its course. Its injury usually occurs at the C6–C7 level, where its course is behind the carotid artery and anterior to the vertebral artery [35]. Injuries resulting in hematoma are more common after blind technique or fluoroscopy-guided procedures. USG during the CSB can help visualize the inferior thyroidal artery anterior to the prevertebral fascia. Thus, the US guidance technique may have advantages over the blind technique and fluoroscopy-guided CSB. Kapral et al. reported the incidence of hematoma formation as 25% (3 of 12 patients) with the blind technique, with no hematoma formation with the USG technique [23].

The incidence of anatomic variations of the vertebral artery is high, resulting in accidental injury and severe complications. It is reported that only 93% of vertebral arteries enter the transverse foramen at the C6 level; the remaining 7% have abnormal variations during entrance to the transverse foramen [5, 6]. The abnormal variations were mostly at C5 and could be seen at the C3, C4, and C7 levels. Thus, preprocedural scanning is highly recommended for evaluating vascular structures and planning the needle pathway to prevent potentially dangerous complications [5, 6].

### Temporary Paralysis of the Recurrent Laryngeal Nerve

The recurrent laryngeal nerve is medial and slightly anterior to the sympathetic chain [1]. When the injection is suprafascial but not subfacial as recommended for a better caudal spread, the spread of the drug is usually cephalad, medial, and anterior which can result in paralysis of the recurrent laryngeal nerve. Therefore, this approach increases the risk of hoarseness due to unilateral vocal cord paralysis.

### Thyroid Gland Injury

The needle pathway is through the thyroid gland in the blind, fluoroscopic-guided, and anterior approach to USG techniques for CSB. USG may be helpful to define a needle pathway avoiding the thyroid gland, such as in the lateral approach to CSB, or may aid in recognizing early complications such as hematoma [34, 36]. Narouze pointed out the significance of thyroid gland injury and hematoma formation related to damage to the inferior thyroid artery [35].

### Esophageal Injury

The esophageal injury can result in serious complications, including esophagitis and mediastinitis [5]. The esophagus can be visualized by ultrasound, and an injury can be prevented during the CSB [42]. The esophagus shows a variable course at the C6 vertebra and cricoid cartilage levels. In a study, Bhatia et al. reported the position of the esophagus lateral to the airway in 50% and 74% of the subjects at C6 and C7 levels, respectively [5]. The esophagus has an oval shape with an irregular lumen secondary to mucosal folds, a characteristic appearance under ultrasound view. The esophagus can be separated from other structures in the neck by observing peristaltic movements when the patient is asked to swallow. The esophagus is more prone to injury in blind or fluoroscopy-guided CSB. When USG-CSB is used, the esophagus is typically not in the needle pathway. However, it is recommended to visualize the esophagus in the preliminary scanning, especially when performing a left-sided CSB, as the esophagus mostly deviates to the left of the trachea (50–70%). In a study, Narouze et al. pointed out that US guidance can help avoid soft tissue structures and prevent esophageal puncture [36].

### Mediastinitis and Mediastinal Emphysema

USG is suggested for avoiding esophageal penetration and its complications. Mediastinitis and mediastinal emphysema can result from an esophageal injury that occurs unintentionally during SGB [36]. As the pharyngoesophageal diverticulum (Zenker diverticulum) is primarily asymptomatic and unrecognized, the presence of the diverticulum is a risk for esophageal penetration and its complications [36].

Needle penetration through the esophagus can lead to bacterial contamination of the needle, resulting in mediastinitis. As mentioned earlier, care should be taken to recognize the esophagus, especially during the left-sided CSB, to avoid injury to the esophagus.

### Other Infectious Complications

Other possible infectious complications after CSB may include local abscess, cellulitis, and osteitis of the vertebral body or transverse process [11].

### Bilateral Injections Should Be Avoided

At the C7 level, the stellate ganglion is posterior to the pleura, with a risk of pneumothorax [1, 34]. USG may help visualize the apex of the pleura and lungs to avoid pneumothorax. Bilateral CSB should be avoided to prevent possible bilateral complications such as recurrent laryngeal nerve block, diaphragmatic block, or pneumothorax. In addition, there is also a possibility of hemodynamic compromise due to anesthetic spread to the vagus nerve or carotid baroreceptors [27].

## Literature on Effectiveness and Safety of US-Guided CSB in Pain Management

Kapral et al. suggested that USG-SGB may improve the procedure's safety while allowing the visualization of the local anesthetic depot. Visualizing the local anesthetic spread might help clinicians avoid side effects as well as typical complications of CSB [23].

In a study, Imani et al. aimed to compare and evaluate the effectiveness of CSB under both fluoroscopy and ultrasound guidance for the management of CRPS [19]. According to the results, Imani et al. reported that USG-CSB is a safer and more effective method with lower complication risk.

In an observational study, Bhatia et al. reported that the USG-CSB via lateral (in-plane) approach at the C6 level could be a safer option for CSB [5]. They performed US scanning of the neck at the C6 and C7 levels in 100 adult subjects. The esophagus location was found lateral to the airway in 50% and 74% at C6 and C7 levels, respectively. During the anterior approach, a major vessel was observed in the needle pathway (up to 29% and 43% of patients at the C6 and C7 levels, respectively). Therefore, the lateral approach at the C6 level has the least potential for vascular injury and associated complications. Moreover, the applying lateral approach targets the needle in an area anatomically distant from the esophagus.

Baek et al. aimed to compare the effects of USG-CSB applied at C6 and C7 levels by a lateral approach [4]. USG-CSB was used twice (once at C6 and once at C7) on 30 patients in the study. The researchers compared skin temperature differences before and after CSB and side effects between C6 and C7 groups. They concluded that performing USG-CSB at the C7 level was more effective at elevating skin temperature in the upper extremity than performing the block at the C6 level.

In a recent study, based on the retrospective analysis of 809 USG-CSB in a total of 105 patients with the diagnoses of CRPS and neuropathic pain, the USG-CSB technique was reported to be safer and more effective [3]. The researchers analyzed the data, including volume and type of local anesthetics, pain levels, the skin temperature changes of hands, heart rate, blood pressure, and occurrence of Horner's syndrome or complications. The results indicated that following the USG-CSB series, pain reduction was more significant with a lower complication rate.

Lee et al. aimed to examine the minimal volume of local anesthetic required for effective blockade for USG-CSB [28]. They found that a small volume of 2 ml of local anesthetic may be sufficient for a successful USG-CSB. Hence, the authors recommend 2 ml of local anesthetic for USG-CSB to prevent unwanted adverse effects from CSB. In a similar study, Jung et al. evaluated the optimal volume of local anesthetics needed for a successful USG-CSB [22]. They suggested an optimal volume of local anesthetics (0.2% ropivacaine) as 4 ml for the USG-CSB.

In a study, Higa et al. evaluated retropharyngeal hematoma patients (27 patients) after SGB in the past 40 years [15]. The patient's symptoms were neck pain, dyspnea, neck swelling, and hoarseness. Twenty-one patients (78%) had airway obstruction, and emergency airway management (orotracheal intubation in 17 patients and emergency tracheostomy in 5 patients) was needed. The authors pointed out that significant distortion of the anatomy can lead to difficult airway management. The authors reported one death as a result of failed airway management. Therefore, a retropharyngeal hematoma is a potentially catastrophic complication of CSB.

In a recent study, Chung et al. aimed to investigate the anatomical distribution of injected local anesthetics and the efficacy of USG-CSB using MR imaging [7]. According to data from post-injection MRI, the researchers reported that the local anesthetic injection spread was found to range between the middle section of C5 and the upper section of the T1 vertebra.

## Summary

Ultrasound-guided (USG) visualization of needles, nerves, blood vessels, and soft tissues can assist the interventionalist in real-time needle advancement. Thus, it may prevent inadvertent tissue trauma and intravascular and intraneural injections [13, 34, 36, 43], allow visualization of medication spread, and reduce the local anesthetic dose required to achieve reliable blockade [22, 23, 28]. The lateral (in-plane) approach at the C6 level has the least potential for vascular injury and associated complications [5]. The cervical sympathetic trunk lies entirely subfascial at the C6 level; therefore, subfascial injection (posterior to the prevertebral fascia and anterior to the longus colli muscle) provides a reliable spread of a solution caudally to the stellate ganglion with less risk of complications [12, 13, 41]. Ultrasound guidance can help the clinician apply proper subfascial injection using real-time needle advancement.

## References

1. Abdi S, Zhou Y, Patel N, Saini B, Nelson J. A new and easy technique to block the stellate ganglion. Pain Physician. 2004;7(3):327–31. PMID: 16858470
2. Ateş Y, Asik I, Özgencil E, et al. Evaluation of the longus colli muscle about stellate ganglion block. Reg Anesth Pain Med. 2009;34:219–23.
3. Aleanakian R, Chung BY, Feldmann RE Jr, Benrath J. Effectiveness, safety, and predictive potential in ultrasound-guided stellate ganglion blockades for the treatment of sympathetically maintained pain. Pain Pract. 2020;20(6):626–38. https://doi.org/10.1111/papr.12892. Epub 2020 May 17. PMID: 32255250
4. Baek J, Kim BS, Yu H, Kim H, Lim C, Song SO. Comparison of ultrasound-guided stellate ganglion block at 6th and 7th cervical vertebrae using the lateral Para carotid out-of-plane approach for sympathetic blockade in the upper extremity. Yeungnam Univ J Med. 2018;35(2):199–204. https://doi.org/10.12701/yujm.2018.35.2.199.
5. Bhatia A, Flamer D, Peng PW. Evaluation of sonoanatomy relevant to performing stellate ganglion blocks using anterior and lateral simulated approaches: an observational study. Can J Anaesth. 2012;59(11):1040–7. https://doi.org/10.1007/s12630-012-9779-4. Epub 2012 Sep 6. PMID: 22956268
6. Bruneau M, Cornelius JF, Marneffe V, Triffaux M, George B. Anatomical variations of the V2 segment of the vertebral artery. Neurosurgery. 2006;59(1 Suppl 1):ONS20–4; discussion ONS20-4. https://doi.org/10.1227/01.NEU.0000219931.64378. B5. PMID: 16888547
7. Chung BY, Holfelder C, Feldmann RE Jr, Kleinboehl D, Raum RC, Benrath J. Magnetic resonance imaging validation of medial transthyroid ultrasound-guided stellate ganglion block: a pilot study. Pain Pract. 2021; https://doi.org/10.1111/papr.13085. Epub ahead of print. PMID: 34662468
8. Darabad RR, Kalangara JP, Woodbury A. Case series: cancer-related facial pain treated with stellate ganglion block. Palliat Med Rep. 2020;1(1):290–5. https://doi.org/10.1089/pmr.2020.0042. PMID: 34223488; PMCID: PMC8241335
9. Day M. Sympathetic blocks the evidence. Pain Pract. 2008;8(2):98–109. https://doi.org/10.1111/j.1533--2500.2008.00177.X. Erratum in: Pain Pract 2008 Jul-Aug;18(4):335–6. PMID: 18366465
10. Ding Y, Yao P, Li H, Han Z, Wang S, Hong T, Zhao G. CT-guided stellate ganglion pulsed radiofrequency stimulation for facial and upper limb postherpetic neuralgia. Front Neurosci. 2019;13:170. https://doi.org/10.3389/fnins.2019.00170. PMID: 30906243; PMCID: PMC6418026
11. Elias M. Cervical sympathetic and stellate ganglion blocks. Pain Physician. 2000;3(3):294–304. PMID: 16906187
12. Ghai A, Kaushik T, Kundu ZS, Wadhera S, Wadhera R. Evaluation of new approach to ultrasound guided stellate ganglion block. Saudi J Anaesth. 2016;10(2):161–7. https://doi.org/10.4103/1658-354X.168815. PMID: 27051366; PMCID: PMC4799607
13. Gofeld M, Bhatia A, Abbas S, Ganapathy S, Johnson M. Development and validation of a new technique for ultrasound-guided stellate ganglion block. Reg Anesth Pain Med. 2009;34(5):475–9. https://doi.org/10.1097/AAP.0b013e3181b494de. PMID: 19920422
14. Gungor S, Brar J. Epidural approach to paravertebral thoracic sympathetic block as an alternative to stellate ganglion block: a case report. Medicine (Baltimore). 2018;97(28):e11492. https://doi.org/10.1097/MD.0000000000011492. PMID: 29995814; PMCID: PMC6076206
15. Higa K, Hirata K, Hirota K, Nitahara K, Shono S. Retropharyngeal hematoma after stellate ganglion block: analysis of 27 patients reported in the literature. Anesthesiology. 2006;105:1238–45. https://doi.org/10.1097/00000542-200612000-00024.
16. Hogan QH, Abram SE. Neural blockade for diagnosis and prognosis. A review. Anesthesiology. 1997;86(1):216–41. https://doi.org/10.1097/00000542-199701000-00026.a. PMID: 9009957
17. Hogan QH, Erickson SJ. MR imaging of the stellate ganglion: normal appearance. AJR Am J Roentgenol. 1992;158(3):655–9. https://doi.org/10.2214/ajr.158.3.1739014. Erratum in: AJR Am J Roentgenol 1992 Jun;158(6):1320. PMID: 1739014
18. Honma M, Murakami G, Sato TJ, Namiki A. Spread of injectate during C6 stellate ganglion block and fascial arrangement in the prevertebral region: an experimental study using donated cadavers. Reg Anesth Pain Med. 2000;25(6):573–83. https://doi.org/10.1053/rapm.2000.8935. PMID: 11097663
19. Imani F, Hemati K, Rahimzadeh P, Kazemi MR, Hejazian K. Effectiveness of Stellate Ganglion Block Under Fluoroscopy or Ultrasound Guidance in Upper Extremity CRPS. J Clin Diagn Res. 2016;10(1):UC09–12. https://doi.org/10.7860/JCDR/2016/14476.7035. Epub 2016 Jan 1. PMID: 26894152; PMCID: PMC4740680
20. Jeon Y. Therapeutic potential of stellate ganglion block in orofacial pain: a mini review. J Dent Anesth Pain Med. 2016;16(3):159–63. https://doi.org/10.17245/jdapm.2016.16.3.159. Epub 2016 Sep 30. PMID: 28884148; PMCID: PMC5586552
21. Jones GP, Tripathi SS. Successful use of stellate ganglion block and a new centrally acting analgesic with dual mode of action in a resistant temporomandibular joint pain. BMJ Case Rep. 2014;2014:bcr2013203308. https://doi.org/10.1136/bcr-2013-203308. PMID: 24849638; PMCID: PMC4039930
22. Jung G, Kim BS, Shin KB, Park KB, Kim SY, Song SO. The optimal volume of 0.2% ropivacaine required for an ultrasound-guided stellate ganglion block. Korean J Anesthesiol. 2011;60(3):179–84. https://doi.org/10.4097/kjae.2011.60.3.179.

23. Kapral S, Krafft P, Gosch M, Fleischmann D, Weinstabl C. Ultrasound imaging for stellate ganglion block: direct visualization of puncture site and local anesthetic spread. A pilot study. Reg Anesth. 1995;20(4):323–8. PMID: 7577781
24. Karmakar MK, Soh E, Chee V, Sheah K, editors. Sonoanatomy relevant for ultrasound-guided injections of the cervical spine, Atlas of sonoanatomy for regional anesthesia and pain medicine. New York: McGraw Hill; 2018.
25. Kim ED, Yoo WJ, Kim YN, Park HJ. Ultrasound-guided pulsed radiofrequency treatment of the cervical sympathetic chain for complex regional pain syndrome. Medicine. 2017;96(1):e5856. https://doi.org/10.1097/MD.0000000000005856.
26. Kim H, Song SO, Jung G. A lateral paracarotid approach for ultrasound-guided stellate ganglion block with a linear probe. J Anesth. 2017;31(3):458–62. https://doi.org/10.1007/s00540-017-2354-y. Epub 2017 Apr 28. PMID: 28455598
27. Korbe S, Udoji EN, Ness TJ, Udoji MA. Ultrasound-guided interventional procedures for chronic pain management. Pain Manag. 2015;5(6):465–82. https://doi.org/10.2217/pmt.15.46.
28. Lee MH, Kim KY, Song JH, Jung HJ, Lim HK, Lee DI, et al. Minimal volume of local anesthetic required for an ultrasound guided SGB. Pain Med. 2012;13(11):1381–8. https://doi.org/10.1111/j.1526-4637.2012.01495.x.
29. Lipov EG, Joshi JR, Sanders S, et al. Effects of stellate-ganglion block on hot flushes and night awakenings in survivors of breast cancer: a pilot study. Lancet Oncol. 2008;9:523Y532.
30. Lipov EG, Lipov S, Joshi JR, Santucci VD, Slavin KV, Beck Vigue SG. Stellate ganglion block may relieve hot flashes by interrupting the sympathetic nervous system. Med Hypotheses. 2007;69:758Y763.
31. Liu Q, Zhong Q, Tang G, Ye L. Ultrasound-guided stellate ganglion block for central post-stroke pain: a case report and review. J Pain Res. 2020;13:461–4. https://doi.org/10.2147/JPR.S236812. PMID: 32161490; PMCID: PMC7049743
32. Moon S, Lee J, Jeon Y. Bilateral stellate ganglion block for migraine: a case report. Medicine (Baltimore). 2020;99(18):e20023. https://doi.org/10.1097/MD.0000000000020023.
33. Mulvaney SW, McLean B, de Leeuw J. The use of stellate ganglion block in the treatment of panic/anxiety symptoms with combat-related post-traumatic stress disorder; preliminary results of long-term follow-up: a case series. Pain Pract. 2010;10:359Y365.
34. Narouze S. Ultrasound-guided stellate ganglion block: safety and efficacy. Curr Pain Headache Rep. 2014;18(6):424. https://doi.org/10.1007/s11916-014-0424-5. PMID: 24760493
35. Narouze S. Beware of the "serpentine" inferior thyroid artery while performing stellate ganglion block. Anest Analg. 2009;109:289Y290.
36. Narouze S, Vydyanathan A, Patel N. Ultrasound-guided stellate ganglion block successfully prevented esophageal puncture. Pain Physician. 2007;10(6):747–52. PMID: 17987096
37. Peng PW. Ultrasound for pain medicine intervention: a practical guide. Vol 1: Peripheral structures. Philip Peng education series; California; iBook, Apple Inc; April 30, 2013
38. Rastogi S, Tripathi S. Cardiac arrest following stellate ganglion block performed under ultrasound guidance. Anaesthesia. 2010;65(10):1042. https://doi.org/10.1111/j.1365-2044.2010.06487.x. PMID: 21198471
39. Shankar H, Simhan S. Transient neuronal injury followed by intravascular injection during an ultrasound guided stellate ganglion block. Anesth Pain Med. 2013;2(3):134–7. https://doi.org/10.5812/aapm.7823. Epub 2013 Jan 1. PMID: 24244924; PMCID: PMC3821125
40. Shanthanna H. Utility of stellate ganglion block in atypical facial pain: a case report and consideration of its possible mechanisms. Case Rep Med. 2013;2013:293826. https://doi.org/10.1155/2013/293826. Epub 2013 Aug 26. PMID: 24065993; PMCID: PMC3770018
41. Shibata Y, Yoshihiro F, Toru K. A new approach of ultrasound-guided stellate ganglion block. Anesth Analg. 2007;105(2):550–1. https://doi.org/10.1213/01.ane.0000265691.02963.a4.
42. Siegenthaler A, Mlekusch S, Schliessbach J, Curatolo M, Eichenberger U. Ultrasound imaging to estimate risk of esophageal and vascular puncture after conventional stellate ganglion block. Reg Anesth Pain Med. 2012;37(2):224–7. https://doi.org/10.1097/AAP.0b013e31823d40fe. PMID: 22157739
43. Soneji N, Peng PW. Ultrasound-guided pain interventions – a review of techniques for peripheral nerves. Korean J Pain. 2013;26(2):111–24. https://doi.org/10.3344/kjp.2013.26.2.111.
44. Takanami I, Abiko T, Koizumi S. Life-threatening airway obstruction due to retropharyngeal and cervicomediastinal hematomas following stellate ganglion block. Thorac Cardiovasc Surg. 2009;57(5):311–2. https://doi.org/10.1055/s-2008-1038845. Epub 2009 Jul 23. PMID: 19629898
45. Uchida T, Nakao S, Morimoto M, Iwamoto T. Serious cervical hematoma after stellate ganglion block. J Anesth. 2015;29(2):321. https://doi.org/10.1007/s00540-014-1914-7. Epub 2014 Sep 26. PMID: 25256578
46. Wang S, Zhu Y. A case report of stellate ganglion block in the treatment of epileptic pain. Medicine (Baltimore). 2017;96(6):e6044. https://doi.org/10.1097/MD.0000000000006044. PMID: 28178147; PMCID: PMC5313004
47. Wei K, Feldmann RE Jr, Brascher AK, Benrath J. Ultrasound-guided stellate ganglion blocks combined with pharmacological and occupational therapy in complex regional pain syndrome (CRPS): a pilot case series ad interim. Pain Med. 2014;15(12):2120–7. https://doi.org/10.1111/pme.12473. PMID: 25537318

48. Wen S, Chen L, Wang TH, Dong L, Zhu ZQ, Xiong LL. The efficacy of ultrasound-guided stellate ganglion block in alleviating postoperative pain and ventricular arrhythmias and its application prospects. Neurol Sci. 2021;42(8):3121–33. https://doi.org/10.1007/s10072-021-05300-4. Epub 2021 May 18. PMID: 34008041
49. Yoo SD, Jung SS, Kim HS, Yun DH, Kim DH, Chon J, Hong DW. Efficacy of ultrasonography guided stellate ganglion blockade in the stroke patients with complex regional pain syndrome. Ann Rehabil Med. 2012;36(5):633–9. https://doi.org/10.5535/arm.2012.36.5.633. Epub 2012 Oct 31. PMID: 23185727; PMCID: PMC3503938

# Glossopharyngeal Nerve Block

Ayhan Cömert, Halil Cihan Köse, Ela Cömert,
Taylan Akkaya, and Selin Güven Köse

## Anatomy

The glossopharyngeal nerve (GPN) is the ninth cranial nerve, which carries predominantly sensory, efferent motor, and preganglionic parasympathetic fibers. Originating from the medulla oblongata, the GPN exits the skull through the jugular foramen along with the vagus and spinal accessory nerves, which is where the tympanic nerve branches off to provide parasympathetic innervation to the parotid gland. Descending between the internal carotid artery (ICA) and internal jugular vein (IJV), the GPN courses medially behind the styloid process, starting to course away from the vagus nerve and proceeding toward its terminal branches. The anatomical course of GPN and its relations with neurovascular anatomical structures were demonstrated in a cadaver neck region (Fig. 1). The extracranial course of the GPN is along the posterior surface of the stylopharyngeus muscle. The styloid process extends inferiorly and anteriorly from the inferior surface of the temporal bone, serving as the point of origin for the styloglossus, stylohyoid, and stylopharyngeus muscles. The length of the styloid process varies among individuals, and the line that connects the gonial angle and the mastoid crosses over the tip of the styloid process. A 3D CT (computed tomography) image was presented here; the patient first applied to the pain clinic with glossopharyngeal neuralgia symptoms, and its 3D CT images demonstrated a long styloid process (Fig. 2).

The nerve follows a path along the lateral surface, eventually exiting through the gap between the superior and middle constrictors and reaching the posterior surface of the tongue near the palatine tonsil [1].

The GPN provides sensory innervation to the upper pharynx, vallecula, the anterior surface of the epiglottis, soft palate, the inner surface of the tympanic membrane, tonsils, and the posterior third of the tongue. Visceral afferent fibers transmit signals originating from the taste buds located in the posterior third of the tongue. Additionally, the GPN carries motor fibers to the stylopharyngeus muscle, which is responsible for elevating the pharynx and larynx [1, 2]. Typically, in the pharynx, the GPN follows a path that curves anteriorly around the stylopharyngeus muscle.

A. Cömert (✉)
Ankara University School of Medicine,
Department of Anatomy, Ankara, Turkey

H. C. Köse · S. G. Köse
Kocaeli City Hospital, Department of Pain Medicine,
Kocaeli, Turkey

E. Cömert
Kırıkkale University Faculty of Medicine,
Department of Otorhinolaryngology,
Head and Neck Surgery, Kırıkkale, Turkey

T. Akkaya
Etlik City Hospital, Department of Anaesthesia and
Pain Medicine, Ankara, Turkey



T. Akkaya, A. Cömert (eds.), *Practical Guide for Pain Interventions: Head and Neck Sonoanatomy*,
https://doi.org/10.1007/978-3-031-88773-4_14

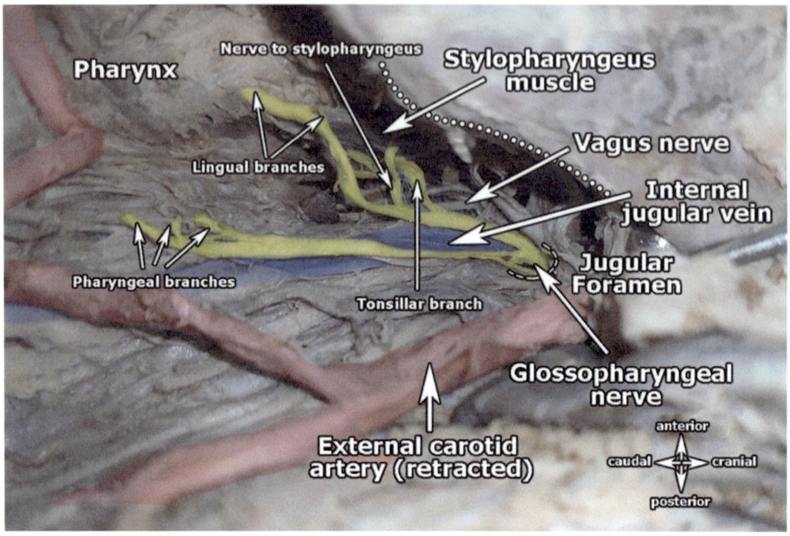


**Fig. 1** The anatomical course of GPN, its branches, and its relations with neurovascular anatomical structures was demonstrated in the left cadaver neck region (dotted lines show a lower margin of ramus of mandible)

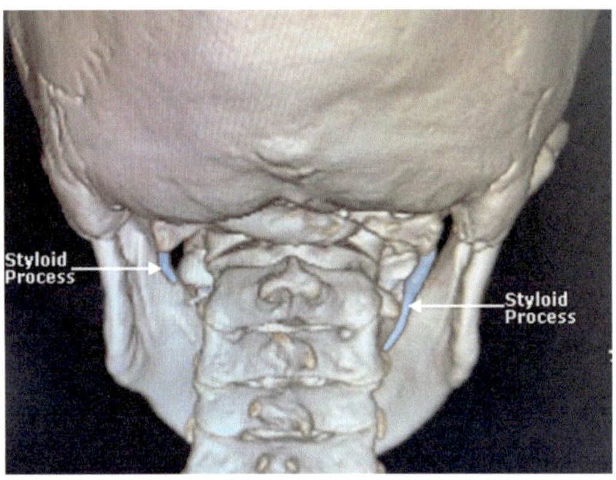


**Fig. 2** 3D CT images demonstrated long styloid process in a patient with Eagle's syndrome

However, a study has reported instances where the GPN instead penetrates through the stylopharyngeus muscle [3]. The carotid sinus nerve, also known as Herring's nerve, is a small branch originating from the GPN. It provides innervation to both the carotid sinus and the carotid body. Parasympathetic fibers of the GPN originate from the inferior salivatory nucleus, which provides fibers to the parotid gland. The GPN and the vagus nerve are closely positioned until they diverge at the midpoint of the styloid process. Notably, there have been reported cases of glossopharyngeal neuralgia paroxysms accompanied by bradycardia and asystole. This occurrence can be attributed to the close connections between the vagus nerve and the GPN [4, 5].

## Indications

Clinically, a GPN block can be performed for a variety of diagnostic and therapeutic procedures.

***Diagnostic:*** The diagnostic GPN block plays an important role in assessing head and facial pain. Its purpose is to confirm the clinical diagnosis of glossopharyngeal neuralgia or Eagle's syndrome. Additionally, the GPN block is performed to predict the response to radiofrequency or neurolysis in intractable glossopharyngeal neuralgia and cancer-related pain syndromes.

***Therapeutic:*** The GPN block is performed to reduce the gag reflex and decrease discomfort during interventions such as bronchoscopy, gastroscopy, and transesophageal echocardiography, as well as for dental procedures in the posterior regions of the oral cavity (e.g., preparation of cavities or crowns in posterior teeth, extraction of third molars).

- Awake endotracheal intubation.
- Acute pain (e.g., post-tonsillectomy, abscess drainage).

- Chronic malignant pain in the oropharynx, the tongue, and the upper airway (e.g., orofacial cancer, pharyngeal cancer).
- Carotid sinus syndrome.
- Hiccups (Singultus).
- Patients who are poor candidates for microvascular decompression [6–10].
- Glossopharyngeal neuralgia.

## Glossopharyngeal Neuralgia

Glossopharyngeal neuralgia is a rare chronic pain syndrome in the sensory distribution of the GPN, comprising approximately 1% of cranial neuralgias. The incidence is approximately 0.7/100000. Typically, it begins after the sixth decade, and the prevalence of glossopharyngeal neuralgia is similar between males and females. As per ICHD-3 (International Classification of Headache Disease-3) classification, it is characterized by episodic, unilateral, severe, sharp shocks of electricity and stabbing transient pain experienced in the ear, tongue base, tonsillar fossa, or angle of the jaw. It also involves the pharyngeal and auricular branches of the vagus nerve. The pain usually lasts for seconds to 2 min and follows a relapsing pattern. Patients may rarely present with arrhythmias and syncope. Pain in glossopharyngeal neuralgia is commonly triggered by swallowing, talking, coughing, chewing, or sensory stimulation such as salty, cold, or acidic foods [11, 12].

In approximately 1–2% of cases, cardiovascular symptoms such as bradycardia, hypotension, and even cardiac arrest can occur during the attacks of glossopharyngeal neuralgia. This connection between glossopharyngeal neuralgia and cardiac symptoms may be attributed to the close association between the glossopharyngeal nerve and the vagus nerve.

Glossopharyngeal neuralgia and trigeminal neuralgia can have similar symptoms, such as facial and jaw pain triggered by similar mechanical and sensory mechanisms. Distinguishing between the two syndromes can be challenging, especially when the pain is located near the tragus or deep within the jaw angle. However, glossopharyngeal neuralgia is relatively uncommon compared to trigeminal neuralgia, although there have been reported cases of both conditions occurring together. Besides, glossopharyngeal neuralgia is more common on the left side, while trigeminal neuralgia is more common on the right side. To differentiate between the two causes, a diagnostic interventional block can be valuable in glossopharyngeal neuralgia diagnosis [13, 14].

Essential or idiopathic glossopharyngeal neuralgia refers to a condition in which the underlying cause or etiology is unknown. The anatomical pathway of the GPN and its associated connections elucidate the symptoms observed in secondary causes of glossopharyngeal neuralgia. Vascular compression of the nerve roots has been the most common pathophysiology of glossopharyngeal neuralgia, leading to demyelination and ephaptic communication. Other secondary causes include demyelinating and inflammatory diseases, oropharyngeal cancers, intracranial tumors, cervical malformations, intraoral and peritonsillar infections, and Eagle's syndrome.

Eagle's syndrome is a rare clinical condition characterized by pain in the anterolateral neck. It occurs when the styloid process becomes elongated, exerting pressure on the GPN, resulting in glossopharyngeal entrapment neuropathy and orofacial pain. Additionally, the elongated styloid process can compress the ICA, leading to carotidynia and neck pain. Typically, the styloid process is considered elongated if its length exceeds 4 cm [15].

The diagnosis of glossopharyngeal neuralgia is mainly clinical, and imaging techniques are performed to determine potential causes of nerve compression. The clinical diagnosis is confirmed by the GPN block. Generally, once medical treatments including anticonvulsants, antidepressants, and analgesics have failed, GPN block with a local anesthetic, neurolysis techniques, radiofrequency ablation, or surgical options are recommended [16].

## Glossopharyngeal Nerve Block Techniques

The GPN block has been performed using topical, intraoral, and peristyloid (percutaneous) approaches. The topical technique may be challenging in patients with limited mouth opening and carries the risk of local anesthetic toxicity. Moreover, this approach is also typically short-acting, and its penetration is limited, primarily affecting the mucosa while the deeper structures maintain sensitivity [17, 18]. In terms of providing a comprehensive block of the GPN, the invasive intraoral and peristyloid approaches are considered more effective. However, these approaches have a risk of injuring or unintentionally injecting into vascular structures such as the carotid artery and the IJV [19]. Therefore, it is crucial to carefully consider the potential risks, including vessel puncture, local anesthetic toxicity, and the possibility of upper airway obstruction when performing these blocks [20, 21]. Additionally, the peristyloid GPN block can inadvertently affect the closely adjacent vagus nerve, resulting in bilateral use of this technique being excessively risky [22].

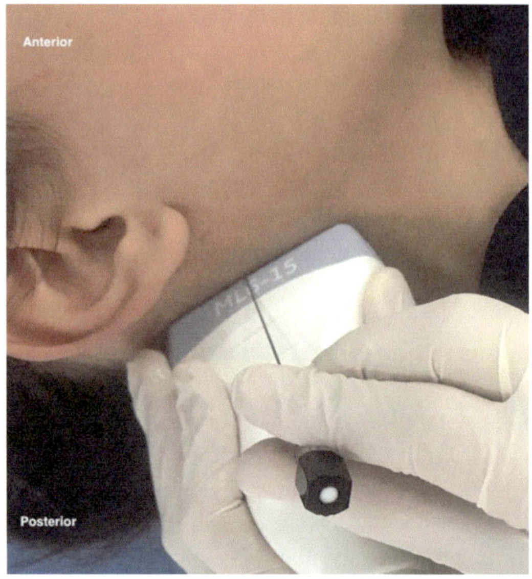


**Fig. 3** Transducer placement for GPN block

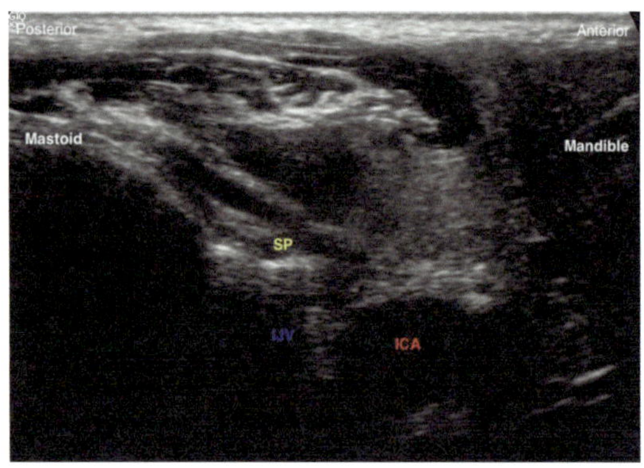


**Fig. 4** Sono-anatomic view of GPN block. SP Spinous process, ICA Internal carotid artery, IJV Internal jugular vein

## Ultrasound (US)-Guided GPN Block

For the procedure, the patient is positioned laterally or supine, with the head rotated slightly away from the affected side. Following the process of sterile cleaning and draping, a subcutaneous local anesthetic was performed. The area over the mastoid process is scanned using a linear probe to locate the mastoid and the mandibular angle. A linear probe is positioned in a transverse oblique orientation between the mastoid and the angle of the mandible, just below the earlobe (Fig. 3). A small hyperechoic shadow, styloid process, is seen medial to the mastoid process. Subsequently, color Doppler is performed to identify the ICA and the IJV mixed blood flow signals below or behind the styloid process. Using an out-of-plane approach, the needle is inserted superior to the probe until it reaches the styloid process (Fig. 4). Then it is slowly withdrawn and directed posteriorly. A solution of 2–3 ml is injected under real-time sonography to allow continuous monitoring of the dissemination of the injectate once a negative aspiration for blood or cerebrospinal fluid is confirmed.

Identifying the styloid process can be challenging due to the presence of bony artifacts from the mandible medially and the mastoid process laterally. In such cases, the ICA is commonly utilized as the primary landmark and is tracked upwards until just below the earlobe. At this level, the carotid artery is situated deep and medial to the styloid process. The needle is administered posteriorly and superficially to the carotid artery even if the styloid process is not visualized clearly [10].

## Complications

Considering the proximity of the GPN to vital vessels and other cranial nerves, the GPN blockade should be performed with standardized monitoring and access to resuscitation equipment. Vascular injury and hematoma can occur from an unintentional puncture of the ICA or IJV. Accidental intravascular injection may result in convulsions or cardiac arrest. Dysphagia may occur due to the blockade of the motor innervation of the stylopharyngeus muscle. Dysphonia owing to paralyzed vocal cords can result from vagus nerve blockade, along with bradycardia, asystole, reflex tachycardia, syncope, and bradycardia. Temporary weakness of the trapezius muscle can result from blockade of the spinal accessory nerve, while blockade of the hypoglossal nerve can lead to temporary weakness of the tongue. Infection is a rare possibility with an aseptic technique, but it becomes an issue in immunocompromised cancer patients [23, 24].

## Literature Review

Currently, there are different approaches for US-guided GPN blocks. The US-guided technique described by Azman et al. involves blocking the GPN distally, depositing local anesthetic into the distal parapharyngeal space, away from the immediate vicinity of high-risk collateral structures [25]. This technique is safer in terms of operative risk as the target is further away from the ICA and IJV compared to the other two methods; however, the target is lower than that of the GPN trunk, resulting in diminished efficacy in the auricular branch. Several studies have reported the effectiveness of distal GPN block in oropharyngeal carcinoma [26–28].

Another method is the US-guided longitudinal axis cervical internal arteriovenous surface block, which targets the GPN trunk at the level of the styloid process or ICA and IJV [29].

In a randomized-controlled study, Sundaram et al. compared the effectiveness of landmark and US-guided GPN blocks in Eagle's syndrome [30]. In the US-guided technique, the target was posterior to the ICA in the submandibular region. If vessels were found in the posterior part of the ICA, they placed the needle tip at different targets. Among the patients, the needle tip was positioned posterior to the ICA in 56% of cases, superior to the ICA in 16% of cases, medial to the ICA in 20% of cases, and between the ICA and IJV in the remaining 8% of cases. They reported that a US-guided GPN block with 1.5 ml of 0.5% ropivacaine and 20 mg of methylprednisolone injected posterior to the ICA in the submandibular region provides better pain relief for at least a week compared with an extraoral landmark technique when three weekly consecutive blocks are given.

In a retrospective study, Liu et al. have shown the effectiveness and safety of US-guided GPN block via the styloid process for primary glossopharyngeal neuralgia. In this transverse axis block of the GPN via the styloid pathway, they used a low-frequency convex probe since the linear probe needs a wide contact area. They claimed that using a convex probe provides scanning of the lower part of the styloid process; therefore, the ICA and IJV under the styloid process can be clearly identified [31].

## Recommendations

Due to its proximity of the GPN to the IJV and ICA, special care should be taken to prevent vascular injury or inadvertent intravascular injection. The vagus, spinal accessory, and hypoglossal nerves also are in proximity to the GPN. While unintentional blocking of these nerves might not be entirely preventable, the risk can be reduced by administering a lower volume of medications. The possibility of bradycardia due to the presence of the carotid sinus nerve requires special caution. Considering the circulatory system side effects, it is necessary to allow the patient to rest for a minimum of 30 min after the procedure.

## References


1. Thomas K, Minutello K, Das JM. Neuroanatomy, cranial nerve 9 (Glossopharyngeal). In: StatPearls. Treasure Island: StatPearls Publishing LLC; 2022.
2. Bedder MD. Glossopharyngeal nerve. In: Hahn, editor. Regional anesthesia. St. Louis: Mosby; 1996. p. 75–9.
3. Sakamoto Y. Morphological features of the glossopharyngeal nerve in the peripharyngeal space, the oropharynx, and the tongue. Anat Rec (Hoboken). 2019;302(4):630–8.
4. Rushton JG, Stevens JC, Miller RH. Glossopharyngeal (vagoglossopharyngeal) neuralgia. Arch Neurol. 1981;38:201–5.
5. Tubbs RS, Mortazavi MM, Loukas M, Shoja MM, Cohen-Gadol AA. Intraoperative and anatomical descriptions of intracranial connections between the glossopharyngeal and vagus nerves: clinical implications. J Neurosurg. 2011;115(1):179–81.
6. Shin JH, Herrera SR, Eboli P, Aydin S, Eskandar EH, Slavin KV. Entrapment of the glossopharyngeal nerve in patients with Eagle syndrome: surgical technique and outcomes in a series of 5 patients. J Neurosurg. 2009;111:1226–30.
7. Costantinides F, Vidoni G, Bodin C, Di Lenarda R. Eagle's syndrome: signs and symptoms. Cranio. 2013;31(1):56–60.
8. Caron H. Control of pain in the head and neck. Otolaryngol Clin N Am. 1981;14:631–52.
9. Shapshay SM, Scott RM, McCann CF, Stoelting I. Pain control in advanced and recurrent head and neck cancer. Otolaryngol Clin N Am. 1980;13(3):551–60.
10. Narouze SN. Glossopharyngeal nerve block. In: Narouze SN, editor. Interventional management of head and face pain. New York: Springer; 2014.
11. Rozen TD. Trigeminal neuralgia and glossopharyngeal neuralgia. Neurol Clin. 2004;22:185–206.
12. Katusic S, Williams DB, Beard CM, et al. Incidence and clinical features of glossopharyngeal neuralgia, Rochester, Minnesota, 1945–1984. Neuroepidemiology. 1991;10(5–6):266–75.
13. Chien GCC, McCormick Z. Glossopharyngeal neuralgia. In: Pope J, Deer T, editors. Treatment of chronic pain conditions. New York: Springer; 2017.
14. Soh KB. The glossopharyngeal nerve, glossopharyngeal neuralgia, and the Eagle's syndrome – current concepts and management. Singapore Med J. 1999;40:659–65.
15. Blumenfeld A, Nikolskaya G. Glossopharyngeal neuralgia. Curr Pain Headache Rep. 2013;17(7):343.
16. Park JS, Ahn YH. Glossopharyngeal neuralgia. J Korean Neurosurg Soc. 2023;66(1):12–23.
17. Rosenberg PH, Heinonen J, Takasaki M. Lidocaine concentration in blood after topical anaesthesia of the upper respiratory tract. Acta Anaesthesiol Scand. 1980;24:125–8.
18. Giordano D, Panini A, Pernice C, Raso MG, Barbieri V. Neurologic toxicity of lidocaine during awake intubation in a patient with tongue base abscess. Case report. Am J Otolaryngol. 2014;35:62–5.
19. Brown DL. Atlas of regional anesthesia. Philadelphia: Saunders; 2010.
20. Pani N, Kumar RS. Regional & topical anaesthesia of upper airways. Indian J Anaesth. 2009;53:641–8.
21. Bean-Lijewski JD. Glossopharyngeal nerve block for pain relief after pediatric tonsillectomy: retrospective analysis and two cases of life-threatening upper airway obstruction from an interrupted trial. Anesth Analg. 1997;84:1232–8.
22. Waldman SD. Styloid process injection. In: Atlas of pain management injection techniques. Philadelphia: Saunders Elsevier; 2013.
23. Jackman C. Head and neck: glossopharyngeal, superior laryngeal, transtracheal block. In: Banik RK, editor. Anesthesiology in-training exam review. Cham: Springer; 2022.
24. Fukui H. Glossopharyngeal nerve block. In: Ohseto K, Uchino H, Iida H, editors. Nerve blockade and interventional therapy. Tokyo: Springer; 2019.
25. Ažman J, StoparPintaric T, Cvetko E, Vlassakov K. Ultrasound guided glossopharyngeal nerve block: a cadaver and a volunteer sonoanatomy study. Reg Anesth Pain Med. 2017;42(2):252–8.
26. Sirohiya P, Kumar V, Yadav P, Bharti SJ. Ultrasound-guided glossopharyngeal nerve block at pharyngeal wall level in a patient with carcinoma tongue. Indian J Palliat Care. 2020;26(01):140–1.
27. Manoharan D, Bharati SJ, Yadav MK. A novel technique of ultrasound-guided glossopharyngeal nerve block to relieve cancer pain. Saudi J Anaesth. 2019;13(03):279–80.
28. Yadav MK, Pulappadi VP, Singh VP, Bharati SJ, Bagga B. Ultrasound-guided glossopharyngeal nerve block-A new paradigm in pain management. J Clin Interv Radiol ISVIR. 2022;07:122.
29. Bedder MD, Lindsay D. Glossopharyngeal nerve block using ultrasound guidance: a case report of a new technique. Reg Anesth. 1989;14(6):304–7.
30. Sundaram S, Punj J. Randomized controlled trial comparing landmark and ultrasound-guided glossopharyngeal nerve in eagle syndrome. Pain Med. 2020;21(6):1208–15.
31. Liu Q, Zhong Q, Tang G, He G. Ultrasound-guided glossopharyngeal nerve block via the styloid process for glossopharyngeal neuralgia: a retrospective study. J Pain Res. 2019;12:2503–10.

# Atlantoaxial and Atlantooccipital Joint Injection

Damla Yürük, Umut Kaan Akçay, and Hüseyin Alp Alptekin

Pain that arises from the atlantoaxial (AAJ) and atlantooccipital joint (AOJ) causes occipitocervical pain syndrome, which is increasingly recognized. The literature that guides the diagnosis and management of pain from AAJ and AOJ is limited and includes a few studies. We aim to review the current information about the pain arising from AAJ and AOJ and also present an ultrasound-guided injection technique.

## Relevant Anatomy

The first two atypical cervical vertebrae (atlas and axis) create AAJ and AOJ. The atlas is a circular-shaped vertebra that articulates with the cranium on it via the lateral mass. It articulates with the axis through its bilateral condyles below. The atlas lacks the spinous process and vertebral body that are found in other cervical vertebrae. The axis has a characteristic projection called the dens of the axis. This structure extends upward from the anterior of the axis. Other features of the axis are the superior articular process, bifid spinous process, and bilateral transverse foramen.

*AOJ* is an ellipsoid-type joint between the superior articular facets of the atlas and the occipital condyle of the occipital bone. It provides the ability for the head to nod forward and backward by flexion and extension to the head. It is quite different from the lower cervical spine; it has no true facet joint, no true posterior articulation, and no classic intervertebral foramina. Its ligaments are the anterior atlantooccipital membrane and posterior atlantooccipital membrane. At the lower edge of the posterior atlantooccipital membrane is an opening for the vertebral artery (VA) and the suboccipital nerve to pass. The C1 spinal nerve (suboccipital nerve) is near the AOJ, exits between the skull and the C1 vertebra, and provides motor innervation to the suboccipital muscles.

*AAJ* is a biaxial synovial joint that can rotate around the pivot point and is located in the upper part of the neck between the atlas and axis. The basic movement of AAJ is the lateral rotation of the skull. AAJ facilitates the movements of the head and neck together with the neck muscles as well as the protection and stabilization of the head, neck, and internal structures. AAJ consists of three different synovial joints—one medial and two lateral. The medial AAJ consists of two ligamentous structures—the ligamentous rings of the atlas and the transverse ligament of the atlas. The two AAJs located laterally are in the plane-type joint class and move in the sliding type. These two joints are unique in that they do not contain an intervertebral disc. The C2 spinal

D. Yürük (✉) · H. A. Alptekin
Etlik City Hospital, Department of Anaesthesia and Pain Clinic, Ankara, Turkey

U. K. Akçay
Ankara University School of Medicine, Department of Anatomy, Ankara, Turkey



T. Akkaya, A. Cömert (eds.), *Practical Guide for Pain Interventions: Head and Neck Sonoanatomy*,
https://doi.org/10.1007/978-3-031-88773-4_15

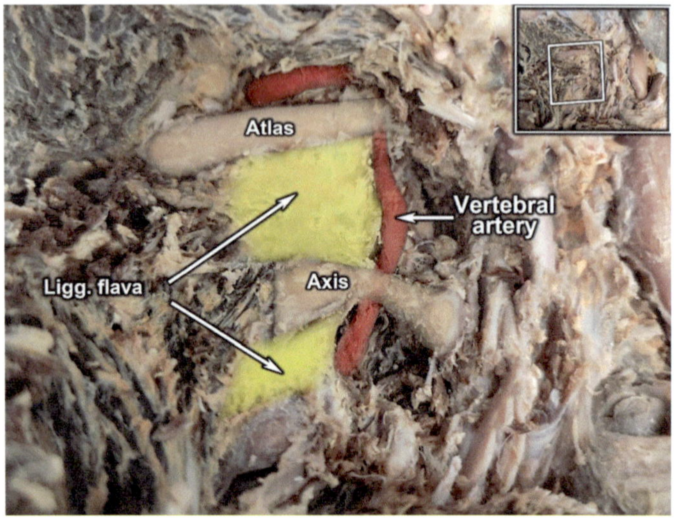


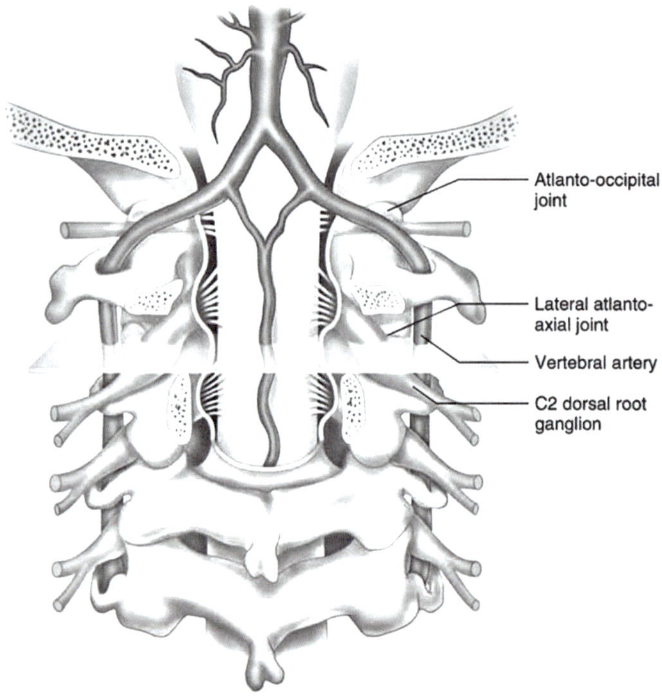


**Fig. 1** View of the course of the vertebral artery at the level of atlantoaxial joint and atlantooccipital joint on a cadaver and schematic picture

nerve is near the AAJ and exits above the C2 vertebra. The C2 dorsal ramus divides into medial (greater occipital nerve) and lateral (supplies the paraspinal musculature) branches. The C2 ventral ramus (lesser occipital nerve) innervates the C1–C2 facet capsule.

*VA* is the most important vascular structure adjacent to AAJ and AOJ. It is one of the vessels feeding the brain together with the internal carotid artery. It passes through the transverse foramen in the transverse process of all cervical vertebrae except the seventh cervical vertebra. It passes through the groove (sometimes canal) for VA on the upper surface of the atlas and comes to the suboccipital triangle. It then passes through the lower border of the posterior atlantooccipital membrane and through the foramen magnum and enters the head. VA ascends from C6 to C1 transverse foramen; as soon as C1 exits the transverse foramen, it turns medially and joins the contralateral VA. During this course, VA travels across the lateral one-third of the AAJ and the medial one-third of the AOJ (Fig. 1).

## Clinical Presentation

The unique anatomy of the AAJ and AOJ makes them susceptible to shear and compression forces. AAJ and AOJ traumatized by acceleration/deceleration injuries constitute 10–30% of all cervical spine injuries, and 20% are fatal [1]. Also can be damaged by arthritis, and the most common cervical spine joints that are affected in patients with rheumatoid arthritis (RA) are the AAJ and AOJ [2]. Although the inflammation responsible for pain caused by trauma or arthritis tends to decrease with conservative treatments in the acute period, it may progress to a chronic stage. Inflammation of the AAJ results in neck disability, nerve root compression, and finally spinal cord compression.

The patient suffering pain arising from the AOJ and AAJ will frequently complain of upper neck pain, occipital, suboccipital, and preauricular headache. It is exacerbated with lateral range of motion, flexion, and extension of the upper cervical spine. It is typically unilateral or worse on one side, has a deep, boring, or aching nature, and restricts motion [3]. Patients also tend to have unilateral tenderness on the affected side, which is not associated with sensory changes [4]. In addition to these symptoms, dizziness, sleep disturbance, nausea, and difficulty in concentrating can be seen.

*Common Features of AAJ and AAJ-Induced Pain:*

1. Pain is usually unilateral in the upper neck, occipital, suboccipital, and preauricular regions.
2. Pain has a deep, boring, or aching nature.
3. Pain restricts function, exacerbated by movement of the upper cervical spine.
4. Sensory and motor symptoms rarely accompany with pain.

It has been reported in many articles that AAJ and AOJ are sources of pain. Intra-articular saline applied to the AAJ has been shown to reproduce occipital and postauricular pain in patients with lateral mass arthritis [5]. Pain patterns that were provocated by injections arising from AAJ and AOJ were first reported as a transverse band at the level of the involved joint [6]. But the recent reports have shown that the pattern of pain is more heterogeneous. A study that described pain arising from AOJ reported headache in 14/20 (70%) cases, posterior neck pain (PNP) in 20 cases, and referred pain in 17 (85%) cases [7]. AOJ and AAJ-arising pain coexist with pain from the C2/C3 facet joints, C1, C2, and C3 nerve roots due to the convergence of fibers from these anatomic structures with trigeminal afferent fibers via the trigeminocervical nucleus. Therefore, pain arising from cervical structures supplied by the upper cervical spinal nerves could be perceived in areas innervated by the trigeminal nerves, such as the orbit and the fronto-temporo-parietal region. This convergence explains the overlapping pain symptomatology and heterogeneity in pain patterns.

## Differential Diagnosis

It is difficult for clinicians to diagnose AAJ and AOJ-induced pain based on history and physical examination findings alone. Imaging studies such as radiography, computed tomography (CT), and magnetic resonance (MR) have limitations in the diagnosis of AAJ and AOJ pathology and are usually used to eliminate other lesions [8]. The differential diagnosis for occipitocervical pain is extensive, and many causes in etiology should be ruled out. These include vascular headache (vertebral artery aneurysm, basilar artery spasm), tension headache, Paget disease, myofascial pain, trauma, O–C1 or C2–C3 arthritis, cervical disc herniation, giant cell arteritis, RA, erosive osteoarthritis, intracranial and intraspinal tumors, congenital anomalies (Chiari malformation), and infection [9].

The clinical presentation described above has a positive predictive value of only 60% and cannot be used alone for the diagnosis of AAJ and AOJ pain [5]. In most cases of AOJ and AOJ-induced pain, imaging shows unilateral joint degeneration. Although the degeneration may be bilateral, it is worse on the affected side. However, abnormal findings on imaging studies do not necessarily mean that the joint is painful. Likewise, the absence of abnormal findings does not prevent the joint from being painful. Reduction of pain with local anesthetic injection to AOJ and AAJ confirms the diagnosis in suspected cases.

## Indications for AAJ and AOJ Injection

The intraarticular local anesthetic injection is used to make a definitive diagnosis of pain arising from the AAJ and AOJ. After the diagnosis, intraarticular steroid, which is thought to be short-acting, or radiofrequency lesioning, which is thought to be longer-acting, can be applied for treatment purposes [10, 11].

Absolute indications for arthrodesis of the lateral AAJ and AOJ include intractable pain, myelopathy, and progressive neurologic deficit. The response to intraarticular local anesthetic injection should be evaluated before such an invasive surgery when selecting patients [12].

Cervicogenic headache is pain originating from cervical structures innervated by the upper three cervical spinal nerves. AAJ and AOJ are innervated by the C2 ventral ramus and thus can cause cervicogenic headache, and intra-articular injection can be applied in the treatment [5].

## Ultrasound Technique of AOJ Injection

The patient is placed in the prone position with the patient's cervical spine flexed. A low-frequency (2–5 Hz) curvilinear transducer is placed in the longitudinal position slightly off the midline over the upper cervical vertebra (Fig. 2). VA is identified as it passes through the transverse foramina between the occiput and the atlas. The artery is then traced cranially by slowly moving the transducer in a cranial direction until the VA is seen to turn medially in front of the AOJ (Fig. 3). In most patients, the AOJ can be identified just lateral to the point where the VA turns medially. In an occasional patient, the VA over-

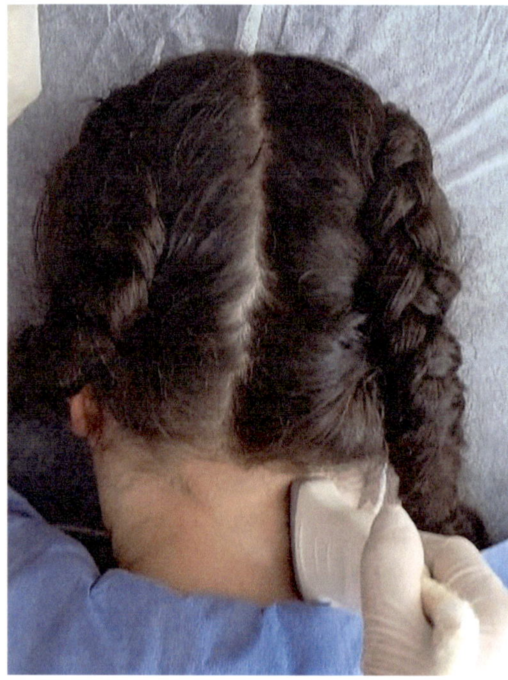

**Fig. 2** Position of patient and ultrasound probe while targeting atlantooccipital joint

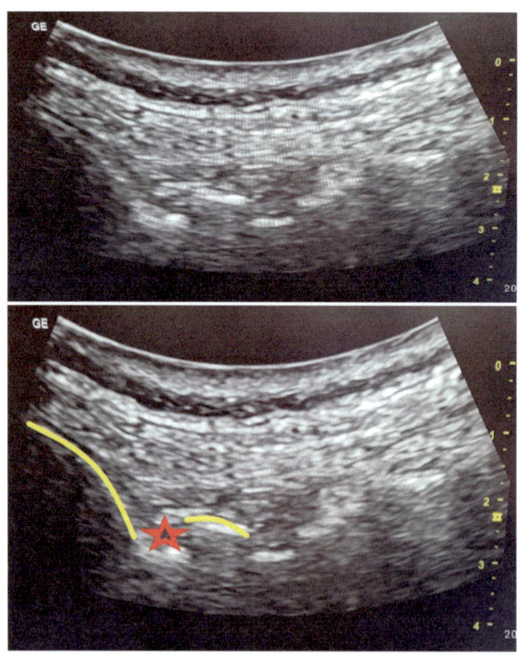


**Fig. 3** Visualization of the occiput and atlas and identification of the vertebral artery between Yellow lines: occiput and C1 lateral mass, red star: vertebral artery

lies the complete extent of the joint as the artery courses from lateral to medial to join the contralateral VA, which makes accessing the insert extremely difficult and insecure.

## Ultrasound Technique of AAJ Injection

The patient is placed in the prone position with the patient's cervical spine flexed. A high-frequency linear transducer is placed in the transverse plane in the midline at the level of the occiput (Fig. 4). The transducer is then slowly moved caudally to identify the C2 vertebral body with a bifid spinous process, making its identification easier. When the C2 vertebra is identified, the transducer is then moved laterally until the exiting C2 nerve root is identified. The transducer is then moved slightly more laterally until the VA is identified. Color Doppler may be used if the VA is not readily apparent. The AAJ should then

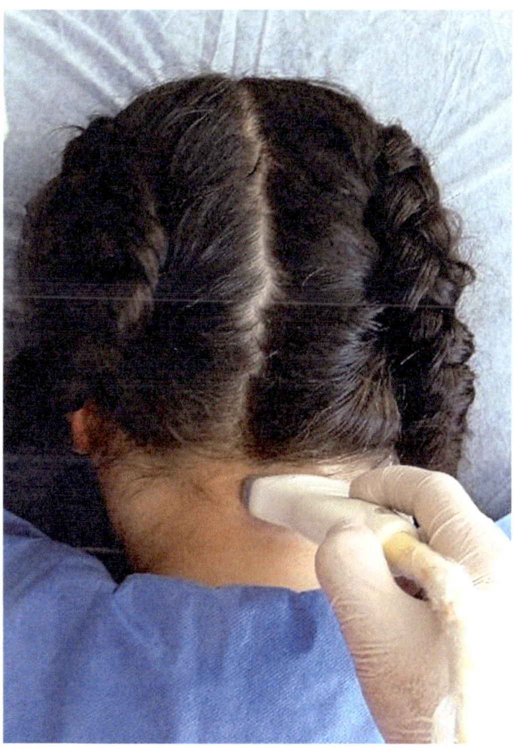

**Fig. 4** Position of patient and ultrasound probe while targeting atlantoaxial joint

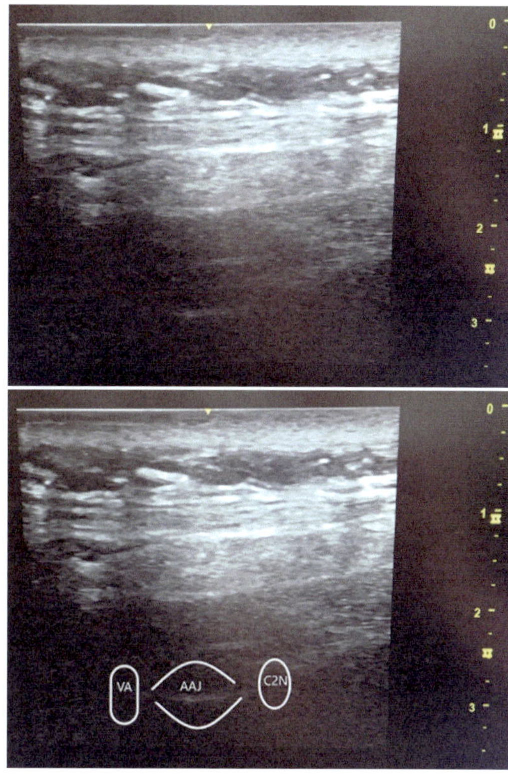


**Fig. 5** Imaging of atlantoaxial joint between C2 root and vertebral artery

be easily identified between the exiting C2 root and the VA (Fig. 5). After the AAJ is revealed in the screenshot, the needle is inserted with the out-of-plane technique into the AAJ without contacting the lateral VA and the medial C2 nerve root.

## Therapeutic Effect of AAJ and AOJ Steroid Injections and Radiofrequency

Hetta et al. reported the efficacy of triamcinolone injection to AAJ in sixty patients with RA who complained of neck pain. Patients were randomized into two groups. Group AAJI ($n = 30$) received an AAJ injection with 1.0 ml of a mixture of 0.5 ml of bupivacaine 0.5% and 0.5 ml of 20 mg of triamcinolone, in addition to oral placebo tablets. Group SS ($n = 30$) received systemic steroids and oral prednisolone tablets, in addition to AAJ injection with 1.0 ml of a mixture of 0.5 ml of bupivacaine 0.5% and 0.5 ml of normal saline solution. There was a significant reduction in the percentage of patients who showed ≥50% reduction of their pain score postoperatively in group AAJI compared with group SS at 1 month and 3 months [13].

Narouze and Gutenberg reported favorable long-term outcomes after both pulsed and thermal radiofrequency lesioning of the lateral AAJ [11]. Halim et al. reported the treatment results of 86 patients, applying 45 V, 2 Hz, and 10 ms for 10 min of pulsed radiofrequency to the lateral C1–2 joint for cervicogenic headache. The percentages of patients who had ≥50% pain relief at 2 months, 6 months, and 1 year were 50% (43/86), 50% (43/86), and 44.2% (38/86), respectively [14].

Busch and Wilson, Dreyfuss et al., and Lee et al. demonstrated the effect of injection of steroid and local anesthetic to the AOJ in patients suffering from headache and neck pain arising from the AOJ [15–17]. Most recently, Shin et al. evaluated the clinical effect of AOJ PRF and compared the effect of PRF to that of intraarticular corticosteroid injection in patients with chronic suboccipital neck pain. Twenty-three patients were divided into one of two groups. Twelve patients received PRF in the IA space of the AOJ (PRF group), and eleven patients received AOJ corticosteroid injection (ICI group). Pain scores were reduced compared to those pretreatment in both groups. Successful pain relief was achieved in 66.7% and 63.6% of patients in the PRF and ICI groups, respectively, and treatment effects continued for at least 6 months [18].

## Complications of AAJ and AOJ Injection

AAJ and AOJ injections have the potential for serious complications, required by appropriately trained physicians under the guidance of imaging modalities (fluoroscopy, ultrasound, CT).

1. *Infection:* Infectious arthritis may occur if the procedure is not performed under sterile conditions. Central nervous system infections are also possible due to the proximity of the joints to the spinal cord and the base of the brain.
2. *VA injection/injury:* It is a serious complication that can cause significant morbidity or mortality. Vascular spread of small amounts of local anesthetic through the VA, regardless of concentration, causes seizures and respiratory arrest.
3. *C1/C2 nerve root and spinal cord injury:* If the needle is guided a few millimeters medially, the dural sheath and neural structures may be damaged. Total spinal block develops when local anesthetic is given in this position.

## Conclusion

AAJ and AOJ may be the source of pain in cervical spine-related traumas, neck pain, headaches in RA patients, and cervicogenic headaches. It is difficult to diagnose clinically and radiologically; injection of local anesthetic into the joint clarifies the diagnosis in many cases. The area is rich in nerves and vessels, which make injections difficult and potentially a source of complications. Interventional procedures should be applied carefully under imaging guidance for patients with a confirmed diagnosis; intra-articular corticosteroids are beneficial in the short and medium term.

## References


1. Olinger C, Bransford R. Upper cervical trauma. Orthop Clin North Am. 2021;52(4):451–79.
2. Wasserman BR, Moskovich R, Razi AE. Rheumatoid arthritis of the cervical spine clinical considerations. Bull NYU Hosp Jt Dis. 2011;69:136–48.
3. Ehni G, Benner B. Occipital neuralgia and the C1-2 arthrosis syndrome. J Neurosurg. 1984;61:961–5.
4. Buraimoh MA, Massie LW, Montgomery DM. Lateral atlantoaxial osteoarthritis: a narrative literature review. Clin Spine Surg. 2017;30(10):433–8.
5. Aprill C, Axinn MJ, Bogduk N. Occipital headaches stemming from the lateral atlanto-axial (C1-2) joint. Cephalalgia. 2002;22:15–22.
6. Dreyfuss P, Michaelsen M, Fletcher D. Atlanto-occipital and lateral atlantoaxial joint pain patterns. Spine. 1994;19:1125–31.
7. Lee DG, Cho YW, Jang SH, Son SM, Kim GJ, Ahn SH. Effectiveness of intra-articular steroid injec-

tion for atlanto-occipital joint pain. Pain Med. 2015;16(6):1077–82.
8. Ogoke BA. The management of atlanto-occipital and atlanto-axial joint pain. Pain Physician. 2000;3:289–93.
9. Cesmebasi A, Muhleman MA, Hulsberg P, et al. Occipital neuralgia: anatomic considerations. Clin Anat. 2015;28:101–8.
10. Narouze SN, Casanova J, Mekhail N. The longitudinal effectiveness of lateral atlanto-axial intra-articular steroid injection in the management of cervicogenic headache. Pain Med. 2007;8:184–8.
11. Narouze SN, Gutenberg L. Radiofrequency denervation of the lateral atlantoaxial joint for the treatment of cervicogenic headache (abstract). Reg Anesth Pain Med. 2007;32:A-8–184.
12. Ghanayem AJ, Leventhal M, Bohlman HH. Osteoarthrosis of the atlantoaxial joints- long term follow up after treatment with arthrodesis. J Bone Joint Surg Am. 1996;78:1300–7.
13. Hetta DF, Elawamy AM, Hassanein MM, Aljohi AS, Hasan RA, Mohammed NAA, Seifeldein GS. Efficacy of atlantoaxial joint glucocorticoid injection in patients with rheumatoid arthritis: a randomized trial. Pain Physician. 2019;22(4):E295–302.
14. Halim W, Chua NH, Vissers KC. Long-term pain relief in patients with cervicogenic headaches after pulsed radiofrequency application into the lateral atlantoaxial (C1-2) joint using an anterolateral approach. Pain Pract. 2010;10(4):267–71.
15. Busch E, Wilson P. Atlanto-occipital and atlanto-axial injections in the treatment of headache and neck pain. Reg Anesth. 1989;14:45.
16. Dreyfuss P, Rogers J, Dreyer S, Fletcher D. Atlanto-occipital joint pain. A report of three cases and description of an intraarticular joint block technique. Reg Anesth. 1994;19:344–51.
17. Lee DG, Cho YW, Jang SH, et al. Effectiveness of intra-articular steroid injection for atlantooccipital joint pain. Pain Med. 2015;16:1077–82.
18. Shin SM, Kwak SG, Lee DG, Chang MC. Clinical effectiveness of intra-articular pulsed radiofrequency compared to intra-articular corticosteroid injection for management of atlanto-occipital joint pain: a prospective randomized controlled pilot study. Spine (Phila Pa 1976). 2018;43(11):741–6.

# Ultrasound-Guided Temporomandibular Injection

Shaw-Gang Shyu, Ming-Yen Hsiao,
and Chueh-Hung Wu

## Anatomy and Function of the TMJ

The TMJs are the paired synovial joints connecting the mandible to the temporal bone. The TMJ is surrounded by a joint capsule and reinforced by temporomandibular ligament (lateral ligament), stylomandibular ligament, and sphenomandibular ligament.

With an articular disk, it forms a complex joint and functions as a hinge joint and a gliding joint. The disc divides TMJ into two compartments, the lower and upper ones. Both compartments are synovial joints. The shape of the disc is biconcave. The superior head of the lateral pterygoid muscle inserts onto the anterior portion of the disc. Both upper and lower compartments do not communicate with each other in regular situations.

The sensory innervation of TMJ is by auriculotemporal (posterior aspect) and masseteric (anterior aspect) branches of the mandibular branch of the trigeminal nerve. The proprioception of lateral pterygoid muscle also provides the sensation, while lateral pterygoid muscle is innervated by the lateral pterygoid nerve, a branch of the mandibular nerve.

The blood supply of TMJ comes mainly from the superficial temporal branch of the external carotid artery (ECA). Other branches of the ECA may also contribute to the blood supply, such as the deep auricular artery, anterior tympanic artery, ascending pharyngeal artery, and maxillary artery.

Bilateral TMJs function together for the movement of the mandible. During mouth opening, the condylar head rotates (as a hinge joint) within the lower compartment of the TMJ, and the entire joint complex (condylar head and articular disc) translates forward and downward (as a gliding joint). This translation produces further opening, while a normal full jaw opening provides an inter-incisor distance of 4–5 cm. Movements of the mandible include elevation, depression, lateral excursions, protrusion, and retrusion.

S.-G. Shyu
Department of Medicine, National Taiwan University Cancer Center, Taipei, Taiwan

M.-Y. Hsiao
Department of Physical Medicine and Rehabilitation, College of Medicine, National Taiwan University, Taipei, Taiwan

Department of Physical Medicine and Rehabilitation, National Taiwan University Hospital, Taipei, Taiwan

C.-H. Wu (✉)
Department of Physical Medicine and Rehabilitation, College of Medicine, National Taiwan University, Taipei, Taiwan

Department of Physical Medicine and Rehabilitation, National Taiwan University Hospital Hsin-Chu Branch, Hsinchu, Taiwan



T. Akkaya, A. Cömert (eds.), *Practical Guide for Pain Interventions: Head and Neck Sonoanatomy*,
https://doi.org/10.1007/978-3-031-88773-4_16

## Indications of Injectional Therapy for TMJ

The TMJ disorder often induces pain around it or radiating pain over the facial and neck region, and sometimes there is intra-articular effusion collection.

1. Arthrocentesis of joint effusion: For symptom relief, synovial fluid analysis, culture, cytology evaluation, etc.
2. Intra-articular injection for anti-inflammation medication, prolotherapy, or hyaluronic acid: Some arthritis, like osteoarthritis, rheumatoid arthritis, psoriatic arthritis, and bruxism-related TMJ disorder, may be treated with intra-articular injection.
3. Peri-articular injection for analgesic intervention of TMJ-related pain, such as reduction for joint dislocation.

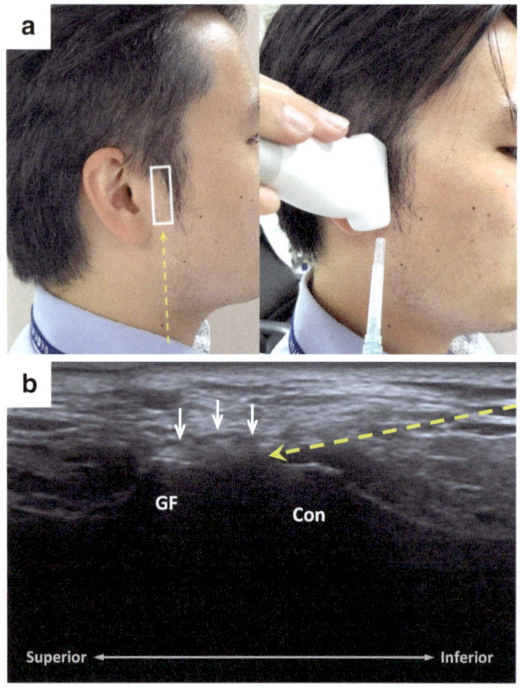


**Fig. 1** Transducer placement (**a**) and sonographic image (**b**) of ultrasound-guided TMJ injection in the coronal plane, in-plane approach. *Con*, mandibular condyle; *GF*, glenoid fossa of temporal bone; arrows, joint capsule; yellow dashed arrow, tract of needle

## Techniques of Ultrasound-Guided TMJ Injection

For ultrasound imaging of TMJ, typically a linear transducer with a frequency of 5–18 Hz is used. A 25-gauge, 1.5-inch needle will usually suffice for TMJ injection. To perform ultrasound-guided TMJ injection, the patient adopts a side-lying position with the lesion side facing up. A generous amount of gel is applied. A standoff pad may be of use in some cases. The injection can be performed in two views: coronal plane and axial plane.

In coronal plane injection, the transducer is placed along the long axis of the mandible ramus (Fig. 1a, b). The mandibular condyle and the glenoid fossa of the temporal bone are identified. An in-plane approach can be performed by inserting the needle caudally beneath the transducer in an inferior-superior direction.[1] The needle is targeted at the joint space at an angle of approximately 30–45° to the skin.

In axial plane injection, the transducer is placed parallel to the Frankfurt horizontal plane (connecting the upper end of the external auditory canal and the lower end of the orbital margin) (Fig. 2a, b). The mandibular condyle, located in the glenoid fossa of the temporal bone, is bounded by the postglenoid tubercle posteriorly and by the articular eminence anteriorly. An out-of-plane approach is suggested for injection in this view [1, 2].

Various anti-inflammatory, lubricant, or irritant medications can be applied in the intra-articular injection of TMJ depending on the disease and treatment purposes. Injection of local anesthetic with or without corticosteroid is commonly used to alleviate pain in inflammatory conditions such as acute arthritis. Hypertonic dextrose, aiming to initiate healing and regenerative response, is often used in osteoarthritis. A randomized controlled trial included 29 patients with chronic TMJ pain and compared the effect of dextrose prolotherapy and lidocaine injection. The dextrose prolotherapy group received three times hypertonic dextrose injection at 1-month

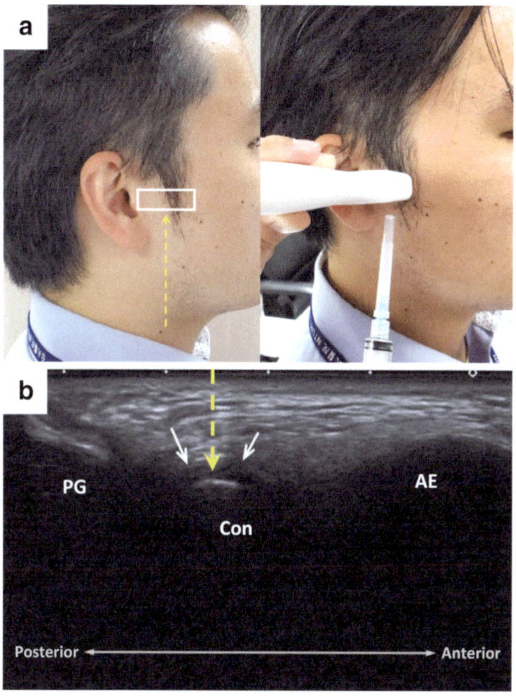


**Fig. 2** Transducer placement (**a**) and sonographic image (**b**) of ultrasound-guided TMJ injection in the axial plane, out-of-plane approach. *AE*, articular eminence of temporal bone; *Con*, mandibular condyle; *PG*, postglenoid tubercle of temporal bone; arrows, joint capsule; yellow dashed arrow, tract of needle

intervals. The pain and maximal jaw opening at 3 months post-injection were similar in both groups, but the dextrose prolotherapy group showed more significant pain relief at 12 months when compared with lidocaine injection [3]. Alternatively, autologous blood or platelet-rich plasma (PRP) can be used in degenerative conditions. The hyaluronic acid injection is another option for treating TMJ dysfunction with clicking or chronic pain. A meta-analysis of six randomized controlled trials concluded that PRP injections provide more pain reduction than placebo injections in osteoarthritis of TMJ at 6 months and 12 months [4]. When compared with hyaluronic acid injections, PRP showed significantly better, though trivial, pain relief at 12 months post-injection.

## Pitfalls and Complications

1. As ultrasound is a dynamic, real-time examination, the images obtained may not be truly coronal or axial.
2. Ultrasound allows visualization of the TMJ structures but does not always allow confirmation of clinical diagnosis based on images. Diagnostic injection may be necessary.
3. Temporary pain or swelling of the TMJ can occur after an intra-articular injection. Steroid flare or infection should be treated accordingly.
4. In some patients, facial muscle weakness, numbness, dizziness, or allergic reactions can be seen.

## References

1. Orhan K, Rozylo-Kalinowska I. Ultrasonography-guided invasive procedures of the temporomandibular joint. Clin Dent Rev. 2021;5:3.
2. Sivri MB, Ozkan Y, Pekiner FN, Gocmen G. Comparison of ultrasound-guided and conventional arthrocentesis of the temporomandibular joint. Br J Oral Maxillofac Surg. 2016;54:677–81.
3. Zarate MA, Frusso RD, Reeves KD, Cheng AL, Rabago D. Dextrose prolotherapy versus lidocaine injection for temporomandibular dysfunction: a pragmatic randomized controlled trial. J Altern Complement Med. 2020;26:1064–73.
4. Li F, Wu C, Sun H, Zhou Q. Effect of platelet-rich plasma injections on pain reduction in patients with temporomandibular joint osteoarthrosis: a meta-analysis of randomized controlled trials. J Oral Facial Pain Headache. 2020;34:149–56.

# Ultrasound-Guided Procedures for Cervical Myofascial Pain

Vincenzo Ricci and Levent Özçakar

## Background

Myofascial pain syndrome (MPS), presenting with multiple symptoms and signs, is very common in the clinical practice of musculoskeletal physicians. The most common pattern is characterized by functional impairment coupled with local and/or referred pain [1, 2]. Myofascial trigger points (MTrPs), i.e., palpable hard nodules housed inside taut bands of skeletal muscles, are considered as the hallmarks of MPS [3]. Direct compression of MTrPs during physical examination usually evokes the pain complained of by the patients [1, 3].

Currently, the diagnosis of MPS is mainly based on clinical findings, i.e., manual identification of the MTrPs within target muscles, coupled with prompt reproduction of local/referred pain induced by compression [3, 4]. In addition to the aforementioned "basic" signs, local twitch response of the MTrPs and release of the taut-band tension induced by manual maneuvers or needling are considered as "advanced" clinical findings that need more experience to be correctly identified [1, 3, 4]. Taking into account the high operator dependence of the manual identification of the MTrPs in daily practice [5], several authors have proposed ultrasound imaging to optimize the management of myofascial pain in the pertinent literature [6, 7]. In this sense, the role of ultrasound imaging appears to be twofold: better identification of the MTrPs [8] and guidance during the interventional procedures [9, 10].

V. Ricci (✉)
Physical and Rehabilitation Medicine Unit, Luigi Sacco University Hospital, ASST Fatebenefratelli-Sacco, Milan, Italy

L. Özçakar
Hacettepe University Medical School, Department of Physical and Rehabilitation Medicine, Ankara, Turkey

## Myofascial Trigger Point Complex

Painful zones in the MPS are characterized by the presence of multiple elements anatomically and functionally connected to each other, also generating the so-called "myofascial trigger point complex" [1, 2]. The taut band of the skeletal muscle shows a main contraction nodule in the central portion and peripheral trigger points at the level of the proximal and distal attachment sites to the bone/periosteum [4]. Within the central trigger point, a variable mixture of normal and abnormal muscle fibers can be observed. The former is characterized by sarcomeres with regular length, and the latter presents a melting pot of shortened and elongated sarcomeres generating multiple contraction knots and distortion of the extracellular matrix [11, 12]. Spatial disorganization of the muscle fibers and endomysium are both considered the main histopathological findings leading to the macroscopic



T. Akkaya, A. Cömert (eds.), *Practical Guide for Pain Interventions: Head and Neck Sonoanatomy*,
https://doi.org/10.1007/978-3-031-88773-4_17

changes of the sonographic texture in the muscle tissue. Magnetic resonance imaging has also confirmed the focal edematous changes— presenting T2 hyperintensity signals—related to the local presence of extra fluids within the micro-cracks of the intercellular scaffold of the skeletal muscle (intercellular edema) [13, 14]. Lastly, high concentrations of glycosaminoglycans within the pathological fissurations of the endomysium are prone to absorb fluids around the contraction knots of the muscle fibers trapping the nociceptive substances [15].

## Sonographic Assessment of the MTrPs

A focal hypoechoic area with heterogeneous inner echotexture is the classical pattern of the myofascial trigger point during the ultrasound examination [6, 7]. Its shape is highly variable—ranging from spherical to elliptical or band-like (Fig. 1) [10]. A wide sonographic tracking of the painful area is usually the first step of the ultrasound assessment to acquire a panoramic view of the different—superficial and deep—muscle layers. The authors suggest slowly shifting the probe over the target area in order to also catch small variations of the muscle echotexture. Moreover, in the presence of sonographic findings compatible with a "potential" trigger point, gentle tiltings of the probe should be performed to avoid fake hypoechogenicity related to the anisotropy artifact. The latter is often related to the (local) presence of multiple muscular fascicles with different spatial orientations [16]. In some patients, peripheral edges of the myofascial trigger point can be blurred and be hardly visible due to connective ramifications within the muscle tissue. In this sense, multiple micro-inclinations of the probe over the hypoechoic nodule can be performed to dynamically optimize its sonographic visibility—the "oscillatory" technique [8]. Color/power Doppler modality must be routinely coupled with the B-mode assessment in order to promptly

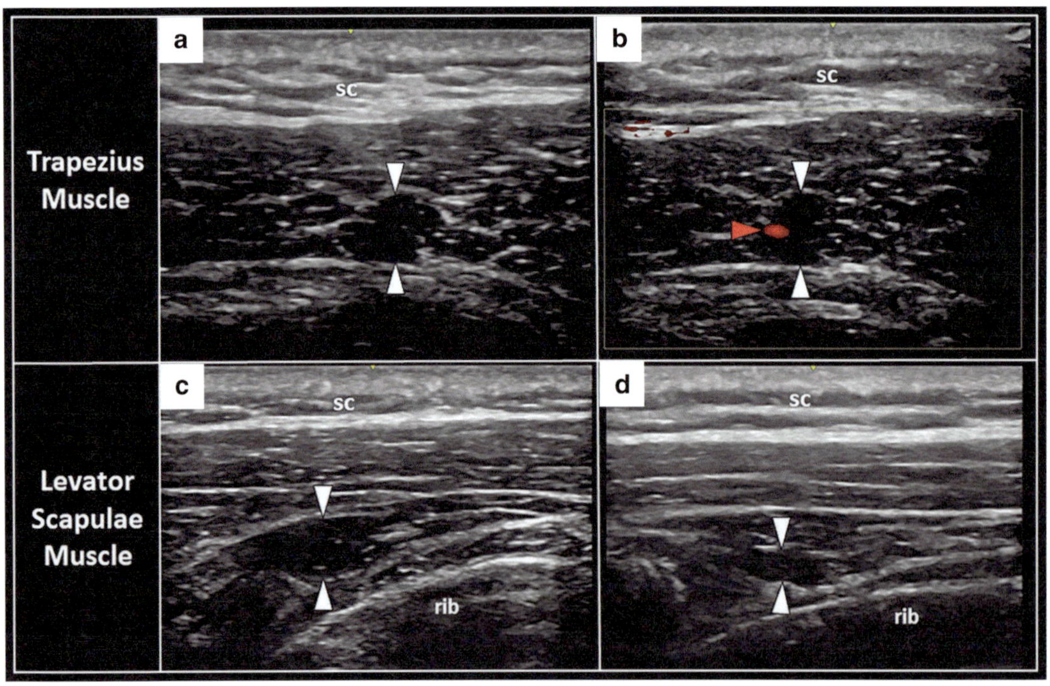


**Fig. 1** Sonography of the myofascial trigger points. A rounded myofascial trigger point (*white arrowheads*) can be observed within the deep portion of the trapezius muscle (**a**). Of note, during the planning phase of the procedure, the peripheral vascular spot (*red arrowhead*) should be considered to better define the needle's pathway (**b**). Likewise, hypoechoic nodules (*white arrowheads*) with different shapes are located at the level of the levator scapulae muscle (**c**, **d**). sc subcutaneous tissue

evaluate (i) the intra-nodular and peri-nodular perfusion pattern (ii) the eventual presence of large vascular structures in close proximity with the myofascial trigger point [10]. Accordingly, an accurate planning phase is crucial in order to define a safe needle pathway, avoiding iatrogenic injury to vital neurovascular structures. Lastly, prompt sono-palpation of the hypoechoic nodule can be performed in an attempt to reproduce the local or referred pain of the patient.

## Ultrasound-Guided Procedures for Cervical Myofascial Pain

Considering the different/multiple pain generators potentially involved in the cervical myofascial pain, three/different types of ultrasound-guided procedures can be performed: (i) injection and/or needling of the myofascial trigger point; (ii) interfascial plane block; and (iii) fascial hydrodissection [8, 17, 18].

In clinical practice, a single intervention or a combination of multiple procedures can be performed in relation to both clinical and ultrasonographic findings. For instance, a single painful myofascial trigger point can be promptly injected under the ultrasound guidance. On the other hand, a large painful zone without the sonographic evidence of hypoechoic nodularities can be managed with other interventional techniques. Likewise, the aforementioned interventional procedures can also be performed with diagnostic purposes in patients with a challenging clinical scenario to better identify the pain generator(s)—i.e., selective diagnostic blocks.

### Injection and/or Needling of the MTP

Based on the above quoted sonographic approach to the MTrPs, it is necessary to clearly define the anatomical location of the hypoechoic nodule and its spatial relation with the surrounding neurovascular structures before performing the procedure [8, 9]. For instance, a deep myofascial trigger point can be located in close proximity of a large artery or lung. As such, extra attention must be paid for planning the intervention. In this sense, the authors suggest considering also alternative therapeutic modalities if the risk to damage vital anatomical structures is high.

A high-frequency linear probe is usually preferred at the level of the cervical spine because it guarantees excellent spatial resolution for superficial anatomical structures [19]. The in-plane technique is generally preferred by the authors to advance the needle within the myofascial trigger point under real-time visualization of the needle's tip throughout the procedure [20]. The approach is largely depending on the spatial location of the painful nodule which differs in each and every patient. For instance, it can be medial to lateral to reach the insertional zone of the rhomboid muscles at the medial border of the scapula, or it can be caudal to cranial targeting the upper fibers of the trapezius muscle [21]. In the authors' experience, the upper fibers of the trapezius muscle and the distal insertional zone of the levator scapulae muscle are the most frequent anatomical sites where the MTrPs are located in clinical practice. Herewith, for sure, painful hypoechoic nodules can be identified in each and every muscle of the cervical spine. Lastly, some tips and tricks should be kept in mind to optimize the clinical efficacy of the ultrasound-guided injection of MTrPs [20]. When the needle's tip is located within the hypoechoic nodule, not "simply" the injection of the mixture but a combination of needling and injection can be simultaneously performed (Fig. 2). Back-and-forward movements of the needle, coupled with fan-like movements of the needle, simultaneously allow greater diffusion of the injection within the pathological area and mechanical disruption of the myofascial trigger point.

### Interfascial Plane Block

As previously mentioned, it is not possible to easily identify a single painful hypoechoic nodule to be injected under ultrasound guidance in each and every patient with myofascial cervical pain [22]. Indeed, multiple hypoechoic nodules involving different muscles or complete absence of focal sonographic findings due to diffuse muscle spasm are some of the possible conditions that can be

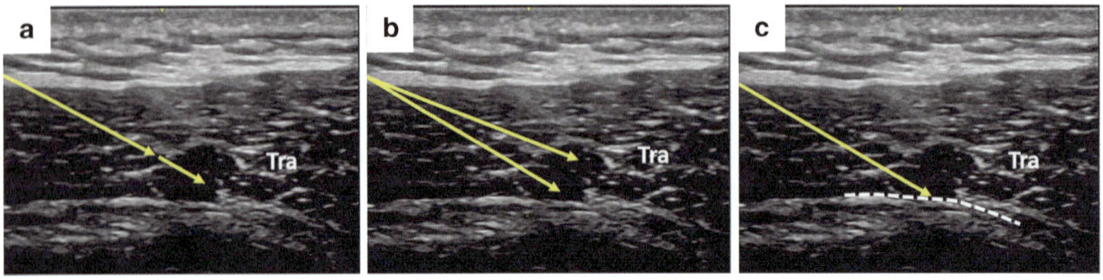


**Fig. 2** Ultrasound-guided treatment of the myofascial trigger point. To perform a multi-step ultrasound-guided procedure, back-and-forward movements (**a**) and fan-shaped movements (**b**) of the needle (*yellow arrow*) can be coupled with hydrodissection of the anatomical interface (*white dotted line*) between the myofascial trigger point and the underlying deep epimysium (**c**). Tra trapezius muscle

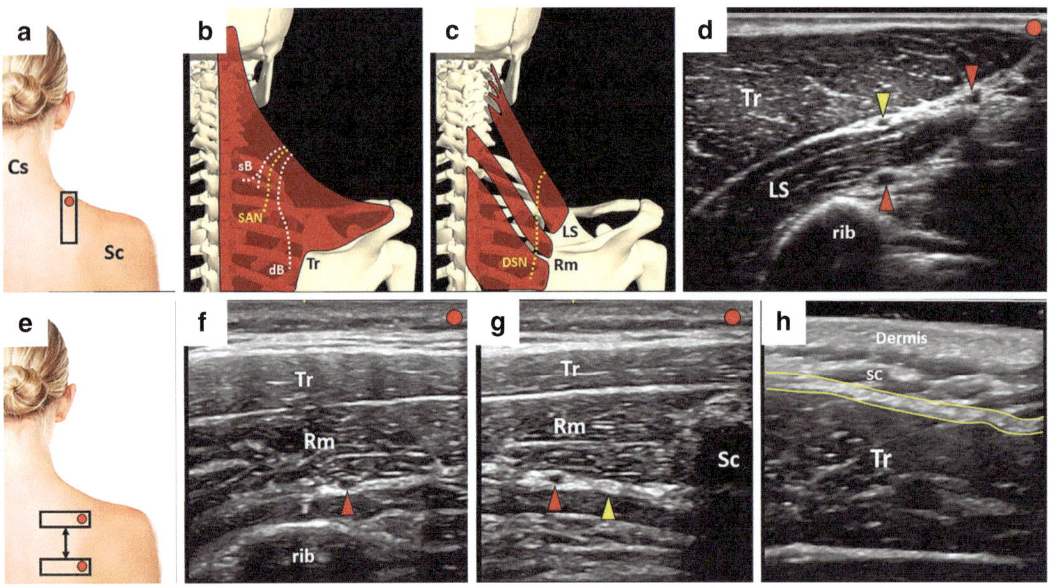


**Fig. 3** Interfascial plane block and fascial hydrodissection. Placing the probe (*black rectangle*) in a longitudinal plane in the anatomical region between the cervical spine (*Cs*) and the scapula (*Sc*) (**a**); the trapezius muscle (*Tr*), superficial (*sB*) and deep (*dB*) branches of the transverse cervical artery, spinal accessory nerve (*SAN*), levator scapulae muscle (*LS*), rhomboid muscles (*Rm*), and the dorsal scapular nerve (*DSN*) can be promptly visualized (**b**, **c**). Of note, vascular (*red arrowheads*) and neural (*yellow arrowhead*) elements can show similar echogenicity during the sonographic examination, whereby color/power Doppler assessment should always be performed to easily differentiate them (**d**). Moreover, a proximal-to-distal or vice versa sonographic tracking (**e**) of the arteries (*red arrowhead*) and/or nerves (*yellow arrowhead*) can be performed (**f**, **g**) in order to better define the safer anatomical site where the interfascial procedure can be performed. The deep fascia (*yellow lines*) of the trapezius muscle (*Tr*) can also be "hydrodissected" layer by layer, considering its potential as a pain generator in the cervical myofascial pain syndrome (**e**). sc subcutaneous tissue

encountered in daily practice [8]. In this sense, ultrasound-guided injection of the interfascial plane can be performed to block peripheral nerve structures physiologically located within this anatomical interface. Yet, within the virtual spaces between the different muscular layers of the cervical spine, many "neural elements" physiologically run as (i) the spinal accessory nerve, (ii) the dorsal scapular nerve, and (iii) the cutaneous branches of the dorsal rami of spinal nerves, which pierce the musculofascial planes of the back to reach the skin [23]. The first two peripheral nerves can be easily identified during the ultrasound examination and be selectively blocked (Fig. 3). However, the tiny

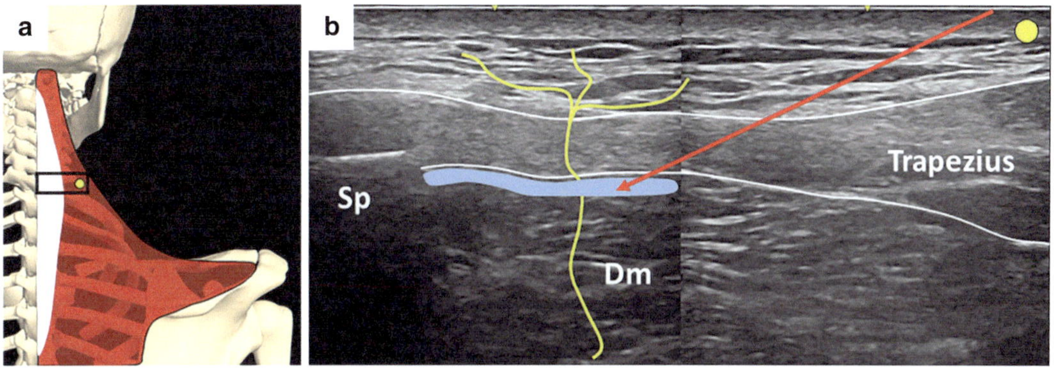


**Fig. 4** Ultrasound-guided block of cutaneous branches of dorsal rami of the spinal nerves. Positioning the probe (*black rectangle*) in the transverse plane (**a**), the needle (*red arrow*) can be advanced—using an in-plane technique and lateral to medial approach—between the fibrous insertion (*white lines*) of the trapezius muscle to the spinous processes (*Sp*) and the deeper muscles (*Dm*) of the cervical spine to block the cutaneous branches (*yellow lines*) of dorsal rami of the spinal nerves (**b**). Light blue pharmacological mixture

terminal divisions of the posterior rami of the spinal nerves directed to the skin are not sonographically visible, and high-volume hydrodissection of fascial planes with anesthetic agents is the best strategy to collectively block them (Fig. 4). In this sense, the spinal accessory nerve can be easily visualized and blocked within the interface between the trapezius and levator scapulae muscles [18, 20]. Likewise, the dorsal scapular nerve can be promptly visualized and blocked within the anatomical plane between rhomboid muscles and the thoracic wall [24].

## Fascial Hydrodissection

The deep fascia is a fibrous structure located between the subcutaneous fat tissue and the muscle [8]. Considering its innervation pattern presenting a high density of free nerve endings, it may play an important role in cervical myofascial pain [25]. In the authors' experience, pain originating from the deep fascia can be coupled with the presence of hypoechoic MTrPs or can represent the main pain generator without other specific sonographic findings [26]. In this sense, it is possible to perform a layer-by-layer hydrodissection of the deep fascia under ultrasound guidance [17] to block the free nerve endings using local anesthetic agents and/or to mechanically dissociate the multiple fibrous layers of the deep fascial structure—to facilitate the so-called "intrafascial gliding" [27]. A long and flexible needle can be used to better "travel" through the multiple layers of the deep fascia, dissociating them with high-volume injection. During both the advancement and retraction phases of the needle, it is possible to slowly release the pharmacological mixture—optimizing the detachment of different layers of the deep fascia.

**Author Disclosures** Conflict of interest: None. No funding was received.

Written permission was obtained from the patients.

## References

1. Gerwin RD. Diagnosis of myofascial pain syndrome. Phys Med Rehabil Clin N Am. 2014;25:341–55.
2. Shah JP, Thaker N, Heimur J, et al. Myofascial trigger points then and now: a historical and scientific perspective. PM&R. 2015;7:746–61.
3. Simons DG. New views of myofascial trigger points: etiology and diagnosis. Arch Phys Med Rehabil. 2008;89:157–9.
4. Simons DG. Review of enigmatic MTrPs as a common cause of enigmatic musculoskeletal pain and dysfunction. J Electromyogr Kinesiol. 2004;14:95–107.
5. Gerwin RD, Shannon S, Hong CZ, et al. Interrater reliability in myofascial trigger point examination. Pain. 1997;69:65–73.
6. Kumbhare DA, Elzibak AH, Noseworthy MD. Assessment of myofascial trigger points using ultrasound. Am J Phys Med Rehabil. 2016;95:72–80.

7. Mazza DF, Boutin RD, Chaudhari AJ. Assessment of myofascial trigger points via imaging: a systematic review. Am J Phys Med Rehabil. 2021;100:1003–14.
8. Ricci V, Ricci C, Gervasoni F, et al. From histo-anatomy to sonography in myofascial pain syndrome: EURO-MUSCULUS/USPRM approach. Am J Phys Med Rehabil. 2022;102:92. https://doi.org/10.1097/PHM.0000000000001975. Epub ahead of print.
9. Kumbhare D, Singh D, Rathbone HA, et al. Ultrasound-guided interventional procedures: myofascial trigger points with structured literature review. Reg Anesth Pain Med. 2017;42:407–12.
10. Sikdar S, Shah JP, Gebreab T, et al. Novel applications of ultrasound technology to visualize and characterize myofascial trigger points and surrounding soft tissue. Arch Phys Med Rehabil. 2009;90:1829–38.
11. Jin F, Guo Y, Wang Z, et al. The pathophysiological nature of sarcomeres in trigger points in patients with myofascial pain syndrome: a preliminary study. Eur J Pain. 2020;24:1968–78.
12. Gerwin RD, Cagnie B, Petrovic M, et al. Foci of segmentally contracted sarcomeres in trapezius muscle biopsy specimens in myalgic and nonmyalgic human subjects: preliminary results. Pain Med. 2020;21:2348–56.
13. Sollmann N, Mathonia N, Weidlich D, et al. Quantitative magnetic resonance imaging of the upper trapezius muscles – assessment of myofascial trigger points in patients with migraine. J Headache Pain. 2019;20:8.
14. Landgraf MN, Ertl-Wagner B, Koerte IK, et al. Alterations in the trapezius muscle in young patients with migraine–a pilot case series with MRI. Eur J Paediatr Neurol. 2015;19:372–6.
15. Margalef R, Sisquella M, Bosque M, et al. Experimental myofascial trigger point creation in rodents. J Appl Physiol. 1985;2019(126):160–9.
16. Wu WT, Chang KV, Hsu YC, et al. Artifacts in musculoskeletal ultrasonography: from physics to clinics. Diagnostics (Basel). 2020;10:645.
17. Wang T, Vahdatinia R, Humbert S, et al. Myofascial injection using fascial layer-specific hydromanipulation technique (FLuSH) and the delineation of multifactorial myofascial pain. Medicina (Kaunas). 2020;56:717.
18. Herbst MK, Sorkin R. Ultrasound-guided spinal accessory nerve block for intractable trapezius pain. Am J Emerg Med. 2022;52(268):e3–268.e7.
19. Ricci V, Abdulsalam AJ, Özçakar L. Ultrasound imaging for dummies: getting oriented among the planes. J Rehabil Med. 2019;51:624–5.
20. Ricci V, Özçakar L. Ultrasound imaging of the upper trapezius muscle for safer myofascial trigger point injections: a case report. Phys Sportsmed. 2019;47:247–8.
21. Ricci V, Özçakar L. Ultrasonographic examination: the "x-factor" in physiatry. Am J Phys Med Rehabil. 2020;99:e131–2.
22. Ricci V, Özçakar L. From "ultrasound imaging" to "ultrasound examination": a needful upgrade in musculoskeletal medicine. Pain Med. 2020;21:1304–6.
23. Domingo T, Blasi J, Casals M, et al. Is interfascial block with ultrasound-guided puncture useful in treatment of myofascial pain of the trapezius muscle? Clin J Pain. 2011;27:297–303.
24. Sultan HE, Younis El-Tantawi GA. Role of dorsal scapular nerve entrapment in unilateral interscapular pain. Arch Phys Med Rehabil. 2013;94:1118–25.
25. Fede C, Pirri C, Fan C, et al. A closer look at the cellular and molecular components of the deep/muscular fasciae. Int J Mol Sci. 2021;22:1411.
26. Pirri C, Ricci V, Stecco C, et al. Clinical and ultrasound examination of the thoracolumbar fascia: the hands and the probe together. Am J Phys Med Rehabil. 2021;100:e157–8.
27. Pavan PG, Stecco A, Stern R, et al. Painful connections: densification versus fibrosis of fascia. Curr Pain Headache Rep. 2014;18:441.

MIX
Papier aus verantwortungsvollen Quellen
Paper from responsible sources
FSC® C105338

If you have any concerns about our products,
you can contact us on
**ProductSafety@springernature.com**

In case Publisher is established outside the EU,
the EU authorized representative is:
**Springer Nature Customer Service Center GmbH**
**Europaplatz 3, 69115 Heidelberg, Germany**

Printed by Libri Plureos GmbH
in Hamburg, Germany